The Thanatology Community and the Needs of the Movement

The Thanatology Community and the Needs of the Movement

Elizabeth J. Clark, PhD, MSW
Austin H. Kutscher, PhD
Editors

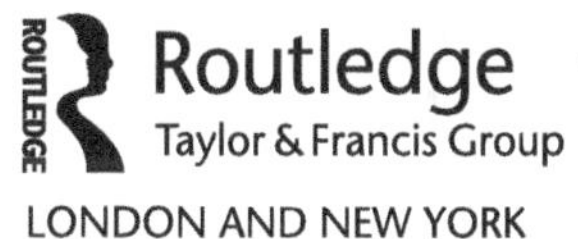

LONDON AND NEW YORK

The Thanatology Community and the Needs of the Movement has also been published as *Loss, Grief & Care*, Volume 6, Number 1, 1992.

First published 1992 by The Haworth Press, Inc.

2 Park Square, Milton Park, Abingdon, Oxon OX14 4RN
711 Third Avenue, New York, NY 10017, USA

Routledge is an imprint of the Taylor & Francis Group, an informa business

First issued in paperback 2016

Library of Congress Cataloging-in-Publication Data

The Thanatology community and the needs of the movement / Elizabeth J. Clark, Austin H. Kutscher, editors.
p. cm.
Includes bibliographical references and index.
1. Death – Social aspects – United States. 2. Thanatology. 3. Death – United States – Psychological aspects. I. Clark, Elizabeth J. 1944- . II. Kutscher, Austin H.
HQ1073.5.U6T47 1992
306.9 – dc20 92-10750
CIP

ISBN 13: 978-1-56024-218-5 (hbk)
ISBN 13: 978-1-138-99012-8 (pbk)

ABOUT THE EDITORS

Elizabeth J. Clark, PhD, MSW, is Director of the Department of Social Work at Albany Medical Center Hospital in Albany, New York, and Associate Professor of Medicine, Division of Medical Oncology, Albany Medical College. She is the Founder and Director of the Social Oncology Network. Dr. Clark has taught courses in thanatology since 1972 at a variety of academic institutions and has published extensively in the field. She is the author of the "Bill of Rights of the Bereaved," and Editor of the journal *Illness, Crises and Loss*. Her research interests include social oncology, quality of life, childhood bereavement, and widowhood. A certified Clinical Sociologist, Dr. Clark is a member of the Academy of Certified Social Workers and is on the Board of Directors of the National Coalition for Cancer Survivorship.

Austin H. Kutscher, PhD, President, The Foundation of Thanatology, New York, New York; Professor of Dentistry (in Psychiatry), Department of Psychiatry, College of Physicians and Surgeons, School of Dental and Oral Surgery, Columbia University, New York, New York.

The Thanatology Community and the Needs of the Movement

The Thanatology Community and the Needs of the Movement

CONTENTS

ALL HAWORTH BOOKS & JOURNALS
ARE PRINTED ON CERTIFIED
ACID-FREE PAPER

The Thanatology Community and the Needs of the Movement

Introduction

Elizabeth J. Clark

In September, 1990, the 1st National Congress of Thanatology was held at Columbia-Presbyterian Medical Center in New York City. Sponsored by the American Institute of Life-Threatening Illness and Loss, A Division of the Foundation of Thanatology, this invitational conference had three main purposes: (1) to bring together leaders in the field of death and bereavement to assess the needs, issues, and problems of the thanatology movement in the United States; (2) to set an agenda for the 1990s; and (3) to lay the groundwork for a national institute or national association of thanatology organizations.

The 148 member Congressional Planning Committee, which spent 2 years on the planning process, chose "The Thanatology Community and the Needs of the Movement" as the theme. The format of the 3 day conference included 14 featured presentations and 15 planning sessions—working group sessions with specific charges. Herman Feifel, editor of the 1959 groundbreaking volume of *The Meaning of Death*, gave the keynote address which is reprinted in this volume.

During the planning process, experts in thanatology were surveyed to ascertain the most important issues facing the thanatology movement. The findings were used as guidelines for determining the Congressional planning sessions. The responses to the survey can be grouped in the 3 areas of general issues, standards, and curricular issues. More specifically, the planning survey listed the following issues as those of greatest concern:

Elizabeth J. Clark, PhD, MSW, Department of Social Work, Albany Medical Center, Albany, NY.

GENERAL ISSUES

- Need for international collaboration
- Need for a clearinghouse for thanatology information
- Establishment of a comprehensive thanatology database
- Lack of coordinated efforts for research and funding
- Need for joint, multidisciplinary research efforts
- Pooling of institutional and association resources
- Better cooperation between academics and practitioners
- Enhanced cooperation to avoid duplication of efforts
- Reduction of interdisciplinary competition
- Policy legislation for issues facing the terminally ill and bereaved
- Increased advocacy for constituent groups
- Enhancement of services for the dying and bereaved
- Communication to public of latest insights and findings from clinical/research/education in thanatology

STANDARDS

- Setting of standards for the field of thanatology
- Certification in general thanatology and in subareas
- Development of educational program guidelines for professional training
- Evaluation of program and clinical interventions

CURRICULAR ISSUES

- Integration of thanatology into professional school curricula
- Integration of bereavement into curriculum as life cycle issue
- Need for death education across the lifespan
- Development of more effective approaches for public education in areas of death and dying
- Public awareness campaigns

The manuscripts included in this volume grew out of the 1st National Congress of Thanatology. Taken as a whole, they do address the major issues facing the thanatology community, and they set a major agenda for the field of thanatology in the coming decade.

REFERENCE

Feifel, Herman (ed.). 1959. *The Meaning of Death*. New York: McGraw-Hill.

The Thanatological Movement: Respice, Adspice, Prospice

Herman Feifel

As to the somewhat baffling title of this manuscript, late last year, in celebration of the 50th anniversary of the Department of Psychology of the City College of New York, I was recognized, along with others, for "outstanding contributions to psychology" and for my "work in the field of thanatology." It happens that the motto of the City College of New York, my undergraduate alma mater, is "Respice, Adspice, Prospice," which translated from the Latin means "regard the past, examine the present, and look toward the future." It struck me that here was an apt triptych to order my remarks. In a certain sense, it reprises a scaffolding I used in 1979 or 1980 to address the annual convention of the Forum for Death Education and Counseling on the nature and future of the modern death movement. This paper can serve as a reliability study of sorts.

So, what I shall do, via broad strokes, is to indicate something about the provenance of the modern death movement, some cardinal clinical and empirical findings emerging thus far from work in the area, and conclude with implications and a perspective concerning challenges and opportunities that face the thanatological community in the next decade or so.

Herman Feifel, PhD, is Chief, Psychology Service, Outpatient Clinic, U.S. Department of Veterans Affairs, Los Angeles, CA.

Keynote address delivered at the First National Congress of Thanatology, Columbia-Presbyterian Medical Center, New York City, September 13, 1990. Preparation of the manuscript was facilitated by a U.S. Department of Veterans Affairs Grant.

PROVENANCE OF THE MODERN DEATH MOVEMENT: RESPICE

Now to the look back part—not, I hope, to return Eurydice to the shades, but rather to avoid a Santayana condemnation. Ancestry of the modern death movement in the Western society dates back to the 17th century when, as a result of the thinking and discoveries of such persons as Descartes, Copernicus, Galileo, and Kepler, individuals started to shift their intellectual inquisitiveness from theology to science, from spiritual mastery over self to physical conquest of nature, and to divorce the cognitive from emotive sphere, mind from body. A prime consequence was transformation of a culture with a religious matrix at its core to one preoccupied with secular pursuits. An aftermath was impoverishment in philosophic and religious creeds, except nominally, with which to transcend death. Death became a "wall," the ultimate personal disaster, rather than a "doorway," and a point in time on the road to eternity. In this discernment, a taboo of considerable degree was placed on death and bereaved persons. Death and it concomitants were sundered off, isolated, and permitted into society only after being properly decontaminated. Another upshot was an increasing fixation on the Cartesian dualism that tended to split the world of science and that of man, and to mute appreciation of wholeness.

Another principal development fueling these perspectives was advent of the industrial revolution with its emphasis on specialization, professionalization, and empowerment of productivity, along with a derogation of minimally contributing members of society. This revolution delivered us from a good deal of physical drudgery but, ironically, resulted in molding many people into impersonal cogs in a big machine, visiting on them a kind of symbolic death. I think part of the violence of our times, not to speak of the irrational and absurd, emanates from these feelings of "psychological" death.

Treatment of the sick was not immune to these unfoldments. Germ orientation and the diseased organ became kingpins of attention for medicine during the latter part of the 19th century. Comprehension of the functioning of human beings became focused mainly within biophysical and chemical frames of reference. Understanding of illness and pathology became linked to an individual's organs rather than to the whole person. This was essentially the regnant state-of-affairs for thanatology in mid-twentieth century.

DEATH RECONSIDERED

Winds of change, however, were blowing. The impact of two World Wars, the Holocaust, the growing prominence of existentialism with its accentuation of death as a philosophical theme, and legacy of the A-bomb with its potential for providing us all with a common epitaph and destroying posterity along with society, began to move matters of meaning, purpose, and temporality, more center-stage. This direction was fortified by a waxing humanism, developments in post-Newtonian physics that increasingly acted on the basis of a field theory, as in Heisenberg's Principle of Indeterminacy. These recognized the observer as part of the observational event, and there was an inextricable interweaving of "fact and interpretation." Also, there was the consequential entrance of the behavioral sciences into the bailiwick of personal conflicts involving moral issues and life choices, and these all coalesced into a view that understanding of behavior must be acquired from human beings, not a mathematical physics model. In this juncture of expanding interest in the pulse of human life and intensified awareness of life's transience, attention to and research in the area of dying, death, and grief began to emerge as an authentic and fertile undertaking.

Additional events animating consciousness of thanatological affairs were reawakened populist, consumerist, and ethnic activities striving to recapture an expanded governance over personal life and greater receptivity for individual will and integrity. In this context, people began demanding a larger shaping role in their own dying and mourning experiences. Closer to home, evolving advances in medical technology were forcing alterations in the character, locus, and time span of dying, economics of dying, raising new ethical perplexities, and challenging the very definition of death—all compelling us to look more steadfastly and systematically at death. In aggregate, there was now an expanded perception and valuing of the influence of death in human conduct, even though some of the occurrences just detailed were escorted by their own innovative modes of death denial.

EARLY YEARS OF THE DEATH MOVEMENT

It might be instructive to review some personal experiences and describe the prevailing climate when I entered on the scene in the early 50s. There was no existing thanatological community or coordinated approach to death at that time. What we did have was heirship to a number of medical, philosophical, sociological, religious, and literary considerations dealing with thanatological concerns. Proper due to their work is manifestly impractical in this synoptic paper. In essence, though, they were as brilliant passing flashes of lightning in a summer sky. Cognoscenti in the field attribute the first organized scientific approach to modern death as being a symposium titled "The Concept of Death and Its Relation to Behavior," which I initiated and chaired, and that was presented at the 1956 annual meeting of the American Psychological Association in Chicago. The symposium provided the groundwork for the 1959 book, *The Meaning of Death*, which I edited, and which most authorities agree was germinal in galvanizing regard for the field and in familiarizing the scholarly community with issues and interests of dying, death, and grief. It seemed to provide a landmark of legitimacy to the newly emerging field. The book itself, however, did not see the light of day without some tribulations. It was rejected originally by both the Oxford University Press and John Wiley before McGraw-Hill took its death-defying dive. Rejection was associated with "no potential market for it," and "this belongs more in the realm of religion." Indeed, even within McGraw-Hill there was an ongoing bet between the Vice President, who favored publishing the book, and the Director of Advertising, who was not so sanguine, whether the book would sell four thousand copies, then a break-even point for the company. Fortunately, the bet was won by the Vice President more than thirty-fold. That same year, 1959, I received what was probably the first research grant awarded to an individual by the National Institute of Mental Health to study attitudes toward death. Despite these initial signs of recognition, numerous scientific Grundys still felt that the topic of death was not appropriate for wissenschaft. *Contemporary Psychology*, for instance, the official book-reviewing journal of the American Psychological Association, rejected considering *The Meaning of Death* because the book had just received a review by *Time* magazine and, hence, had attained its allotted morbid fascination exposure. More telling was the communication that the subject was not germane to genuine scientific inquiry.

The attempt to implement my research mandate relating attitudes toward death and behavior also was beset with manifold vicissitudes and frustrations. Some of the professional personnel with whom I was working told me that at no time did they ever inform patients that they had a serious illness from which they could die. "The one thing you never do," it was emphasized, "is to discuss death with a patient." Along this same line, after a three-month delay in responding to my request for permission to gather data from patients, the chief physician-in-charge of a leading metropolitan hospital finally replied, "Excuse my immoderate delay in answering, but you have to be a staff member," a lack known to him at the inception of our discussion about obtaining patients. The commissioner of hospitals of a major city responded to my request for subjects by saying, "It is not consonant with our policy to set aside patients for this purpose." Then there was the chief research psychiatrist of a prominent medical center who "knew" that the research project would induce what he termed "test toxicity" in the patients, despite already demonstrated results to the contrary.

The realization soon began to sink in that what I was up against were not idiosyncratic personal quirks, the usual administrative vicissitudes, pique, or nonacceptance of an inadequate research design. Rather, it was personal position, bolstered by cultural structuring, that death is a dark symbol not to be stirred—not even touched—an obscenity to be avoided. I must admit to more than passing vagaries about chucking the whole thing. Two things, though, held me to the task. One was my ego. I had made a dent or two, *mirabile dictu*, here and there, using "gameship" of an order that would have warmed Stephen Potter. Second, was my sentiment, albeit occasionally dampened by repeated rejections, that study of the area was important and, come hell or high water, should be implemented. Fortunately, as I have noted, there were exceptions to the situation I have been describing. I did find congenial colleagues and professional personnel who perceived what I was striving to do, acknowledged its importance, and helped me get my work off the ground.

Succeeding years saw a burst of activity in the field. The 1960s and 1970s were characterized by the introduction of workshops and courses on dying, death, and mourning in various universities and professional schools. There were also noteworthy pioneering books by Kastenbaum & Ainsberg (1972), the psychiatrists Eissler (1955), Hinton (1967), Kübler-Ross (1969), Parkes (1972), and Weisman (1972), sociologists Fulton (1965) and Glaser and Strauss (1965), the nurse-sociologist Quint-Benoliel (1967), the philosopher Choron (1963), and cultural anthropologist Gorer (1965), among others. Such pioneering names as Grollman, Jackson, LeShan and Raether also come to mind. It was during this period that Kübler-Ross succeeded in popularizing thanatology among the laity; Cicely Saunders kindled the hospice movement; and Dan Leviton energized the death education sector. Journals such as *OMEGA* (1969; Robert Kastenbaum, editor), *Death Education* (1977; now called *Death Studies*, Hannelore Wass, editor), and the *Journal of Thanatology* (1973; Austin H. Kutscher, editor), came into being. Additionally, a number of scientific and professional associations devoted specifically to thanatological matters were founded. Among the more prominent were the International Work Group on Death, Dying, and Bereavement, the Association for Death Education and Counseling, and the Foundation of Thanatology (now known as the American Institute of Life-Threatening Illness and Loss). Bolstering these groups were several self-help and lay groups for example, Make Today Count (1973), The Society of Compassionate Friends (1969), and widow-to-widow programs sparked by Phyllis Silverman (1969).

CLINICAL PERCEPTIONS AND EMPIRICAL FINDINGS: ADSPICE

What are some leading findings and implications that have surfaced as a result of our labors as a movement?

1. The meaning of death has a shaping power on thinking and behavior at all points in the life span. It is for all seasons and not

just constricted to the terminally ill, suicidal, old, or combat soldier. Children as young as 2-3 years of age already contend with its reality.

2. Cognition of death and fear of death express themselves in dissembling guises and hide in ways of behaving not ordinarily considered to be related to death, for example, insomnia, depression, various psychosomatic symptoms, and certain psychotic manifestations.

3. Fear of death is not a unitary or monolithic feature. Diverse subcomponents are evident, for example, loss of identity, loneliness, going to hell, and having to face the unknown with minimal mastery. Further, significant discrepancies exist in many persons between conscious and nonconscious attitudes toward death. Apprehension about death, for instance, displays itself as a lockstitching phenomenon with little reported fear of death on a verbal conscious level coupled with one of ambivalence on a fantasy or imagery level, and outright negativity on a nonconscious plane. This counterbalance of coexisting avoidance-acceptance of personal death appears to serve powerful adaptational needs. In the face of death, the human mind operates ostensibly on various levels of reality, or finite provinces of meaning, each of which can be somewhat autonomous. This finding seems to have its spur in the stern tradition that assumes we are both terminated by death and yet capable of continuing on beyond death.

4. Grief is not a sign of personal fragility or self-favoring. Rather, it mirrors a normal and profound need most of us have in responding to the death of a significant person in our lives. Moreover, we have learned that a neglected or truncated mourning often may declare itself later on in unsuitable behavior. Some illustrations are school absenteeism and bed-wetting in children, drug abuse and delinquency in adolescents, and promiscuity, suicide, and divergent physical and mental illnesses in adults.

5. Expanded understanding of the many strategies that individuals employ in coping with dying and grief signal that we must guard against promulgating a coercive orthodoxy of how we should die or mourn. Applying Avery Weisman's wise admonition, an "appropriate" dying or mourning is one satisfactory to or, at least, tolerated by the dying person or bereaved survivor, not one so designated by either the helping professions, family and friends, or the

community. Individual differences and esteem for personhood must be our principal guides.

6. Focus has been redirected to the role of the future in steering conduct. How we anticipate and foresee death can govern our "now" in an influential manner. This rediscovery is providing us with a needed antidote to a widespread vogue of being mesmerized by the moment. Indeed, if anything distinguishes human beings as a species, it is our talent to conceptualize a future—and along with it inexorable death. In large measure, this is why the mathematical physics paradigm has never been able to fully encompass the depth and range of human functioning.

7. The movement has sensitized health care professionals and the public to realize that when cure is definitely not in the cards, the provision of care and comfort is just as valid a contribution in meeting real needs of patients and their families. Hospice, of course, is a superb assertion of this understanding.

8. We have underscored the importance of death education in our cultural upbringing as a preparation for living. Our enlightenment has demonstrated its pertinence not only for those in health care who grapple with dying, death, and bereavement, but for all. The call is to alter cultural perspective, not just achieve a palliative interest.

9. We have confirmed the viability and cogency of a transdisciplinary approach in working with dying patients and survivors. Death is too multisplendored and intricate to be the special province of any one discipline.

10. We are helping rehumanize medical treatment of the terminally ill and have forwarded rights of the dying and mourners.

11. Finally, the death movement has performed admirably in elevating collegial and civic consciousness that dying is not just a biological happening, but a human one as well.

IMPLICATIONS FOR THE THANATOLOGICAL COMMUNITY: PROSPICE

What are some mandates for the decade ahead?

1. More scrutiny needs to be devoted to overt and covert connections that may exist between meanings of death and such urgent social issues as abortion, AIDS, euthanasia, and capital punish-

ment, and to such detrimental behaviors as alcoholism, drug abuse, and certain acts of violence. Life-threatening behaviors, after all, involve encounter, in one way or another, with the threat of possible injury or even death to self and others. Spin-offs from such inquiry could tutor us in coping with threat, disaster, loss, and the harassments of old age. In this configuration, the impact of death and deprivation on organizations and institutions, as well as on individuals and families, should be examined more methodically.

2. Another gap which asks for more ordered investigation is the arena of cross-cultural and differing ethnic group attitudes toward death. In a shrinking world, knowledge of such views will be illuminating and guiding.

3. With the movement's progression into adulthood, there has been an inflow into the field of dabblers and dilettantes. This is occasioning a Gresham's Law phenomenon. This is the economic dictum, you remember, wherein inferior money starts to replace good currency. This suggests that the movement address itself, in a more timely manner, to the question of standards for toilers in the thanatological vineyard.

4. We are in want of comprehensive models of death that will incorporate the entire life span into its scope and deliberations. These should build on and amplify the currently influential palliative care prototype. As already emphasized, death's shaping power obtrudes at all age levels, and for the healthy as well as for the sick.

Characteristic of all these assignments should be the intertwining of the clinician's appreciation of individuality and complexity with the researcher's demand for precise and firm documentation. We require comprehension and images that are more fitting to contemporary death and mourning.

We should consider the feasibility of planning for a National Institute of Thanatology similar to those of the National Institute of Mental Health and National Institute on Aging. Such an Institute could promote and catalyze ongoing endeavors, widen the thanatological knowledge base, highpoint priorities, and serve as a resource for funding. It also could arrange for a clearinghouse that would enhance networking and stimulate coordinated efforts.

Life is real and earnest. We, therefore, cannot constrict our offerings, edifying as they may be, to scholarship and learning alone. We shall have to be competent and vigorous participants in helping formulate legislative initiatives and public policy in the thanatological field. Power can be enabling as well as corrupting. This tack is of increasing importance in an era of shrinking financial resources, soaring medical costs, and a burgeoning position that is redefining health care substantially in terms of economics and cost distribution. A bookkeeper mentality is starting to take over. A case in point: Recently the journal *Science* (Morrell, 1990) discussed findings of the highly publicized Oregon State Health Service Commission report studying the rationing of Medicaid dollars by applying cost-benefit ratings to nearly 2,000 medical procedures. A consequential finding arising from use of a mathematical formula to rank-order these procedures in terms of cost-benefit ratios was that such treatments as thumb-sucking and acute headaches ranked higher for care attention than those of cystic fibrosis and AIDS. Immunizations for children's diseases did not even appear on the list. Quality of care for the patient is still receiving lip service, but, all too distressingly, is ofttimes being demoted to "second banana" status. The invitation is to generate a view that will worship the fire, rather than ashes, at the altar. Thanatology's stake is crucial here because many involved in its domain are perceived as tangential, if not outright antithetical, to an assessment that prizes cost-benefit ratios at the expense of humanity.

CONCLUSION

Overall, we are much better situated these days than heretofore to transmit our message. We now speak from a transdisciplinary footing and, in paradoxical fashion, are beneficiaries of a medical technology that is obligating us to look at dying and death more resolutely. As Kastenbaum (1982:161) recently put it, "Death has come a long way from being the skeleton in the closet with Herman Feifel's hand on the doorknob." And, although we are witness to new contemporary denial fantasies of death and are still as "on a darkling plain," receptivity to death has gained entryway into our educational system, stirred mindfulness by the humanities and media, and is becoming a more demanding political and judicial deliberation.

Nevertheless, wherever these new territories lead us, and muffling somewhat my own summons for more public policy engagement, we must remain primarily committed to expanding and deepening our information base so that practice does not outrun knowledge. William James, the eminent psychologist, once stated that he was no lover of disorder but feared to lose the truth by pretensions to wholly possessing it. We must differentiate between performance and public relations—although both plainly have their proper place.

We are currently beholding a new conceptual thrust and praxis in the area spearheaded by immunology, pharmacology, and neurobiology that is augmenting and optimizing treatment intervention. Nevertheless, a caveat is in order. The road ahead should lead to larger horizons without sacrificing gains. This means that as invigorating as the new development is, it must be accompanied by sustained comprehension that the behavioral and social sciences are salient ingredients of an inclusive human biology.

Refinement in the pursuit of our craft, moreover, will not be sufficient unless it is carried out in the framework of healing the humanity of the dying patient and wounded mourner. The humanities, ethics, and the spiritual dimension must be in our ken along with biology and the behavioral and social sciences. Death and grief bring with them preoccupation with a vision of life.

In final analysis, notwithstanding our growing versatility and acknowledgment of political and economic realities, we are, at core, not intrinsically lobbyists, administrators, or politicians, but disciplined, observing, and compassionate helpers. Our ultimate effectiveness will be judged not in terms of the number of laws we succeed in getting passed, but in the number of hearts and souls we touch, the number of lives we help transform. As I have declared in other forums, the death movement and social engineering will clearly never exorcise death of its demonic power and redeem humanity. Death, however, will always be a concern of vernal freshness because it is our birth heritage and destiny. A power which is perhaps greater than the secret of the atom is knowledge of self—of our mortality. In this context, the thanatological community is highpointing values and priorities that undergird the vitality of human response to catastrophe and loss. It is contributing to reconstituting the integrity of our splintered wholeness. And, perhaps more important, it is sensitizing us to our common humanity, all too eroded in the present world. It may be somewhat hyperbolic, but I believe that how we behold death and how we treat the dying and bereaved are prime indicators of a civilizations's intention and target.

Foresight, imagination, and commitment are evident. Convocation of the First National Congress of Thanatology (September, 1990) demonstrated the power of example and perseverance to set others in sympathetic motion. We are aware that, more often than not, progress proceeds from elusive but vital fractions. There is a relevant saying from the Pirke Aboth (Ethics of the Fathers) of the Mishnah (Danby, 1933:449): "It is not thy duty to complete the task, but neither art thou free to desist from it." Our task is to continue extending our grasp of how death can serve life. May we go from strength to strength.

REFERENCES

Choron, J. 1963. *Death and Western Thought*. New York: Collier Books.

Danby, H. 1933. *The Mishnah*. Oxford: Oxford University Press.

Eissler, K.R. 1955. *The Psychiatrist and the Dying Patient*. New York: International Universities Press.

Feifel, H. (Chair). 1956, September. *The Concept of Death and Its Relation to Behavior*. Symposium presented at the meeting of the American Psychological Association, Chicago.

Feifel, H. (ed.). 1959. *The Meaning of Death*. New York: McGraw-Hill.

Fulton, R. (ed.). 1965. *Death and Identity*. New York: Wiley.

Glaser, B.G., and A.L. Strauss. 1965. *Awareness of Dying*. Chicago: Aldine.

Gorer, G. 1965. *Death, Grief, and Mourning*. New York: Doubleday.

Hinton, J. 1967. *Dying*. Baltimore: Penguin Books.

Kastenbaum, R. 1982. New fantasies in the American death system. *Death Education*, 6:155-166.

Kastenbaum, R., and R. Aisenberg. 1972. *The Psychology of Death*. New York: Springer.

Kübler-Ross, E. 1969. *On Death and Dying*. London: Macmillan.

Morrell, V. 1990. News & Comment. *Science*, 249, 468-471.

Parkes, C.M. 1972. *Bereavement: Studies of Grief in Adult Life*. New York: International Universities Press.

Quint-Benoliel, J. 1967. *The Nurse and the Dying Patient*. New York: Macmillan.

Weisman, A.D. 1972. *On Dying and Denying: A Psychiatric Study of Terminality*. New York: McGraw-Hill.

Undervalued Caregiving: A Major Issue for the Thanatology Community

Jeanne Quint Benoliel

Central to the thanatology movement is a concern for the individual—whether that individual be a patient, family member, provider, teacher, or ordinary person facing a life crisis. In nursing this concern has centered on the welfare and well-being of dying patients and their families. It has been reflected in several different phrases—the importance of dying with dignity, the importance of respecting and protecting the autonomy of the dying person, and the provision of family-centered care.

In a real sense, nursing's commitment has been to the importance of personalizing the experience of dying. This focus was central to the Transition Services Model as a framework for the delivery of community-based person-centered services for advanced cancer patients and their families, a model developed by McCorkle and the author at the University of Washington. A central goal of the OTS Model is to support the integrity of the dying person through:

1. Helping that person seek meaning in the experience;
2. Providing help with distressing signs/symptoms;
3. Providing opportunity to bring closure to life.

Provision of this kind of service has been difficult because it does not fit with current policies and practices on what constitutes health care and whether it should be funded. At the heart of the matter is a more central problem—the difficulty of obtaining resources for

Jeanne Quint Benoliel, RN, DNSc, is Professor Emeritus, School of Nursing, University of Washington, Seattle, WA.

caregiving, an activity that is undervalued in current society and is provided often by people marginal to the mainstream of social power—women, minorities, outsiders.

EXPANDING NEEDS FOR CARE

Currently, societal needs for caregiving services are expanding, and for several reasons:

1. An aging population, with the majority of dying patients being over 65 years;
2. People living longer with diseases that in previous centuries would have killed them;
3. Indiscriminant use of lifeprolonging technology has created groups of people who are dependent totally on caregiving services for survival, (e.g., ventilator-dependent children).

Although the demands for caregiving services are growing, caregiving as such is not valued (except in the motherhood sense of the word) and does not have high priority in the allocation of scarce resources for populations in need. The bulk of societal resources for health care continue to be given to recovery-oriented medical treatments, and governmental policies strongly are influenced by a "lifesaving at all costs" ethic. A basic question posed for consideration is:

> Given that dying, like living, is a personal experience, what will it be like in a societal context of limited resources, expanding needs for care, and undervalued caregiving services?

This question is not trivial. At issue for all of us is the power of an attitude that death (like all aspects of the natural world) can be conquered if we humans put enough time, effort, and energy to the task.

If the thanatology community is to move anywhere, there needs to be a recognition of how much the "defeat of death" attitude toward the world influences our ideas, our work, and the settings in which we live. Further, the *medicalization* of major human transition experiences—such as birth, childhood, adolescence, marriage, old age, and death—has contributed to a growing dependence on *experts* for advice on what to do and how to do it more so than self-reliance and personal choice in living though difficult life situations that are part and parcel of the human condition. Also despite the contributions of advanced technologies to improvement in living conditions for many, these same technologies (a) contribute to depersonalization in living for many others; and (b) increase the opportunities for *powerful people* to decide whether some persons whose lives may be viewed as not very valuable should be allowed to die (Hall & Cameron, 1976).

IS AN ECOLOGICALLY-ORIENTED SOCIETY POSSIBLE?

The basic assumption of this paper is that our attitudes toward each other as human beings are influenced by the social environment in which we develop. In current United States society, there is a pervasive emphasis on human beings as *instruments* to be improved, fine-tuned, made thin, or whatever—toward the goal of "living happily ever after." Central to the value system of this country is the concept of individualism, and great importance is attached to personal responsibility for actions taken and competition to become "the best."

There is a need for a shift in orientation away from this self-centered idea of individualism toward a view of the individual as part of a collective enterprise that includes reciprocity, partnerships, and commitments to others and not just competition to make a name for oneself. Individuals need to learn how to give as well as to take, and how to give up so that others may have. How can the thanatology community—as individuals and as a collectivity—engage in activities that foster what Douvan (1977) called the *caring society*? Instead of a society in which neighbors are distanced from one another, she asked:

> What are the conditions that will help people to touch the lives of their neighbors and take responsibility for the security and humaneness of those lives? (p. 27)

She suggested two ways that social policy could be used to foster caring relationships among people:

1. Detecting groups in the community who offer generous caring (e.g., caring for elders at home) and providing modest support through federal funds to reinforce these practices. Potential sources of caring assistance include adolescents, elderly persons, and men and women without other commitments.
2. Implementing programs to develop empathy, commitment, and generosity as human traits to be nurtured and encouraged. Educational institutions and sports activities are key areas for this kind of socialization experience. This perspective should be central to the educational programs preparing people to contribute in fields that have come to be called *Human Services*.

EDUCATION FOR COMMUNAL COMMITMENT

Perhaps one way that we in the thanatology community can contribute (instead of feeling overwhelmed by the enormity of the problem) is to find ways and means to counterbalance the competitive influence of our educational and work environments. In the educational realm, the teacher can make deliberate use of activities that foster sharing and concensual problem-solving. These can include group projects instead of individual papers, a variety of self-learning activities, use of drama as a teaching-learning modality, and course assignments that bring students face-to-face with the human problems that they encounter in the real world of practice.

In teaching a course, "Death Influence in Clinical Practice," across some 20 years, the author has observed the learning value of having out-of-class assignments in a variety of death-related situations. Such "confrontations" with real people in real situations trigger students to reflect on the meaning of death in their own lives and the meaning of death in their work situations. Essentially, I have found that these experiences assist students in their personal growth as human beings faced with the existential realities of death and an uncertain universe.

Of course, to be effective the teacher who wishes to foster communal commitment in students must be willing to make a commitment to the students and to be available to share with them the joys and the pains of learning what it means to be fully human. Education for communal commitment requires reciprocal involvement with students, not the distanced detachment of the expert scholar.

CREATION OF CARING WORK ENVIRONMENTS

Activities to foster the shift of work environments from the current patriarchal, superior-subordinate team orientation toward a view of work as a communal effort is no easy task. One approach to change might be to find ways of incorporating feminist principles of power into the ongoing system of working relationships. Whereas the masculine perspective on power has emphasized use of *power for self*, a feminist perspective views the use of power to enhance *both* self and *other* (Miller, 1976:116-118). To take a new perspective on the meaning of power in human relationships requires examination of some differences in masculine and feminine meanings of the word:

MASCULINE	FEMININE
Results	Process
Prescription	Letting Go
Force	Collectivity
Hierarchy	Unity
Command	Sharing
Polar Opposites	Integration
Use (Exploitation)	Nurturance
Causality	Intuition
Secrecy	Responsibility
Conformity	Diversity

Putting feminist principles of power into action means being oriented to human processes as much as to the outcome of activities, of sharing leadership under different conditions of work, and of using decision-making by consensus (Wheeler & Chinn, 1984). Central to the implementation of feminist principles of power is the creation of social environments in which each participant can grow in terms of personal power and communal participation.

In the thanatology community (whether in our work environments or personal lives) we need to learn to practice empowerment of self and others through: (a) working relationships that are respectful, encouraging, show concern for others, and demonstrate constructive ways of dealing with conflict; and (b) actions that foster collaboration, communication, and support at all levels in the provider community. Empowerment strategies—whether for self-care or care of others—are concerned with self-esteem building in its many forms.

SUMMARY OBSERVATIONS

The heart of caregiving rests in the human relationship between the giver and the receiver of care, and each of us occupies one or the other position at some point in time. Often the situation of caregiving makes heavy demands on the humanity of the caregiver for several reasons: (a) it is centered on the needs of the recipient, and they have primacy; (b) it is labor intensive and demanding of the caregiver's time, energy, and effort; (c) it usually continues for 24 hours of the day; and (d) as a human activity, it is accorded few social rewards in the form of money, position, and prestige (Graham, 1983). People engaged in caregiving need work environments that provide them recognition, nurturance, and opportunities to grow and mature as persons.

This paper has emphasized the importance of reciprocal relationships among providers as well as with the recipients of caregiving services. It argues that the concept of team perpetuates a superior-subordinate work pattern supportive of a patriarchal model of human relationships. It is important for the future of humankind that we in thanatology foster and encourage the creation of caregiving environments in which: (a) the model of delivery is by a *community of colleagues*; (b) the mode of action is through partnerships with patients, families, and other providers; and (c) the mode of relationship is equal and reciprocal (Benoliel, 1990).

To date our work environments have been organized around the valued Western attributes of autonomy and independence, abstract critical thinking, and a morality of rights and justice—representing essentially a masculine perspective. To move toward community in our work environments, we need to find ways of giving credence to what have been called the feminine attributes: intimacy and interdependence, contextual thought, and a morality of responsibility and care for the vulnerable (Belenky, Clinch, Goldberger, and Tarule, 1986).

In the crowded world of the future, human beings will face difficult choices that may include whether or not to set controls on the unrestrained use of biotechnology, how much of social resources to invest in human services such as education and health care, and how to make decisions about the use of lifeprolonging technology. Given the diversity among us, it is essential that we search for ways to communicate across our various differences and to learn to live with death as a part of the human condition—not an enemy to be defeated.

REFERENCES

Belenky, M.F., B.M. Clinch, N.R. Goldberger, and J.M. Tarule. 1986. *Women's Ways of Knowing*. New York: Basic Books.

Benoliel, J.Q. 1990. Healing environments and women in transition: An issue for nursing. In J.J. Fitzpatrick, M.C. England, E. Goodman, and M. Redmon (eds.), *Proceedings of the First and Second Annual Rosemary Ellis Scholars' Retreat* (pp. 131-143). Cleveland: Case Western Reserve University, Frances Payne Bolton School of Nursing.

Douvan, E. 1977. The caring society. *The Center Magazine*, X(2):26-40.

Graham, H. 1983. Caring: A labour of love. In J. Finch & D. Groves (eds.), *A Labour of Love: Women, Work and Caring* (pp. 13-30). London: Routledge & Kegan Paul.

Hall, E., and P. Cameron. 1976. Our failing reverence for live. *Psychology Today*, 19(11):104-113.

Miller, J.B. 1977. *Toward a New Psychology of Women*. Boston: Beacon Press.

Wheeler, C.E., and P.L. Chinn. *Peace & Power: A Handbook of Feminist Process*. Buffalo: Margaretdaughters, Inc.

Educational Needs in Thanatology

Richard R. Ellis

Education is a major industry throughout the world. One of the newer arrivals to education currently is known as *Death Education*. It began in the United States, and is active particularly in North America. As its name might imply, Death Education is a process by which knowledge, skills, and attitudes within the area of death-related topics are imparted to another. Although it draws its life from several disciplines and other sources, it is highly specialized in focus. Nevertheless, more than a dozen different occupational groups currently are engaged in it and the practices deriving from it. It is important to note that while Death Education is ostensibly about death-related topics, it is verifiably about life and living.

Death Education, as we know it in North America today, stems from several roots. Probably the first cogent, systematic examination of those roots appeared when Herman Feifel, a psychologist, published *The Meaning of Death* in 1959. The root system Feifel assembled included the fields of anthropology, art, literature, medicine, philosophy, physiology, psychoanalysis, psychiatry, psychology, and religion. The main tap root was, and is, psychology. From this root system two trunks grew to major proportions.

The substance of the first was a psychological interest in both the inter- and intrapersonal dynamics, the factors, the needs and issues that obtain on the occasion of life-threatening illness, of loss, dying, death, and bereavement. It was a relatively small group of practitioners and scholars who gave it form by fostering its growth, development, and diversification, particularly during the ensuing 15 or so years.

Richard R. Ellis, EdD, is Associate Professor of Applied Psychology, New York University, New York, NY.

As an important example, in 1965, Robert Fulton provided in his *Death and Identity* a sociological perspective which was another part of the root system. This group of pioneers made it possible for the second trunk to sprout.

The substance of the second trunk was education, which took the form of curricular units, courses and seminars, conferences, and so on. During the late 1970s, more and more persons were entering the field and contributing to the viability of this trunk. In 1977, Dr. Feifel revisited *The Meaning of Death* by publishing *New Meanings of Death*. To the former root structure he added business, funerary practices, health education, law, mortuary science, nursing, social work, and thanatology. There was a new plant in the garden: *thanatology*—a term Metchnikoff introduced in 1903 (Kastenbaum & Kastenbaum, 1989), now growing in use as the name of this new interdisciplinary field of practice and study.

Changing the analogue from botany to weaving, psychology and education are the warp and woof of the fabric of Death Education; skeins of detail threads provide image, design, style, and color. Today the fabric comes in a virtually endless variety of choices. For example, the consumer may get a snippet of death when, as a five-year-old, she listens to her mother read E.B. White's classic story for young children, *Charlotte's Web*; or in high school she may get a swatch of "the colors of death" as part of a lesson on art appreciation; or a fragment of "burial practices" in a college course on ancient history; or the full nine yards of "complicated mourning" in a graduate course on bereavement counseling; or, as an adult, she may join a widow's support group in her efforts to shred the shroud of her grief. Even so, the fabric comes cut according to two basic patterns: Death Education for the provider of thanatological services to others, and Death Education for the person learning about thanatological topics. Neither pattern is really independent of the other, but each targets a different audience, holds different objectives, and, although some overlap may occur, addresses different bodies of content.

Individual educators, pre-kindergarten through post-doctoral studies, seem to be the most active group of death educators; individual helping professionals of various persuasions, in a myriad of settings, are another group—as is a lesser number of small teams of those professionals; hundreds of lay persons volunteer their services. With all this activity comes a fracas of issues to be considered.

One very important issue arises from the linkages between the two basic patterns of Death Education. Emotionality may be the most important of these links. For example, feelings of anxiety or fear, guilt or sorrow, pain or relief, and so on, are primary content of Death Education for providers of service. This content, however, can trigger these same feelings in both the death educator and the learner. The issue, then, centers on the preparation of the death educator to handle effectively and appropriately the emotionality present in the educator and in the learner. This is a crucial issue.

This author's position is that until and unless the death educator has, in some meaningful way, faced his or her own mortality and the attendant anxieties, fears, and attitudes, those variables will significantly impede the death educator's functioning. (This applies to other thanatologists as well.) Knowledge about the content of Death Education is a necessary but insufficient condition, to paraphrase the counseling psychologist, Carl Rogers (1957). Thanatological knowledge alone is not enough. The death educator needs knowledge *and* a significant awareness of his or her personal relationship with death. Skills in education and skills in helping others are necessary but insufficient conditions. Skills *and* the awareness of one's personal relationship with death are basic to the effectiveness of a death educator. Attitudes and their corollaries form the key condition. However, it is the triadic presence of the requisite knowledge, skills, and attitudes that provides both the necessary and sufficient conditions.

If this position is valid, then consider that within it lie several challenges to thanatologists. Some questions promptly come to mind:

- How confident can we be that we have identified a body of knowledge sufficient to label as the core content of thanatology?
- What part of a core content should every death educator, regardless of educational level or of target audience, know thoroughly?

- In addition to core knowledge, what body of knowledge should each specialized group (e.g., discipline, field, profession) and each lay group know?
- What educational skills should each death educator possess?
- What clinical skills should each death educator possess?
- What attitudes are most helpful to the process of education? Which are an impediment?
- What are the criteria for success in achieving the desired knowledge, skills, and attitudes? What are the minima?
- Are the ability and the tools to recognize and to assess achievement of knowledge, skills, and attitudes available?

The last two questions relate to objectives and assessment. These are traditional topics among educators involved in curricular decisions. During the 1950s and 60s, the industry of education steered toward the development and application of taxonomies of educational objectives and of behavioral objectives. In 1948, Benjamin Bloom and his colleagues (psychologists and educators) began a project to identify hierarchies of behavior in three domains: cognitive, affective, and psychomotor. In 1956, they published *Taxonomy of Educational Objectives, Handbook I: Cognitive Domain*. The handbook became required reading for almost everyone who was or would be involved in curriculum development. Creating the second handbook revealed even more problems in identifying objectives than did the first, but in 1964, Bloom's group published *Handbook II: Affective Domain*. Problems with the third handbook were greater still, and it has not yet appeared. During the 1960s the buzz words in education were "behavioral objectives," meaning educational goals translated into observable behavior. A typical, and popular, book of the time was Robert Mager's *Preparing Instructional Objectives* (1962). Despite the usefulness of taxonomies and of behavioral objectives in clarifying goals, they did have shortcomings. As thorough as they were, they could not be applied to absolutely every objective.

Following are three examples of problems in application. First, a hierarchy requires placing, i.e., valuing, one construct above another; values from one culture may be quite different from values from other cultures. Second, where in a hierarchy does brotherly love, erotic love, and patriotic love belong? Third, judging the achievement of educational goals by observable behavior rules out attending to and valuing the quick, fleeting, creative insights learners often have as a result of an educational experience. The idea is that appropriateness has a place here; it may be as defeating to adhere strictly to one set of rules for setting objectives (taxonomies, behavioral objectives) as it is to be slave to another (apply little or no specificity to objectives). The successful death educator will employ systems for identifying objectives appropriately and not artificially. For example, common sense informs many in our society that one year of mourning a loved one is the standard, required condition (the behavioral objective). However, informed death educators now know that the period of mourning needed by an individual is highly idiosyncratic.

In general, problems with objectives are related to those of assessment. Obviously the assessor or evaluator needs to know what is to be assessed. Clear objectives might be better assessed than fuzzy objectives; but this may be true only when assessment data can be quantified or when preexisting norms or standards are specified. In Death Education, norms and standards might not yet exist and quantification might not be appropriate for some objectives.

Currently available thanatological knowledge is not yet definitive in every area, but we have learned a substantial amount that provides meaningful insights and guidelines for the death educator. For example, Raphael's (1983) review of research on bereavement is a benchmark of progress.

The *how* of Death Education seems not yet to have received the concerted attention it needs from death educators. The proliferation of Death Education activities has far exceeded the dissemination of thoughtful guidelines for those activities. Most thanatologists can recite at least one horror story of a misfire in the name of Death Education. The incident usually is the result of some person well-intentioned but unguided, supposing but unknowing, and willing but unqualified to enter the arena of Death Education. For readers not knowing an example, here are two—both true; only the names are fictitious.

Ms. Cue, a teacher of fourth grade, read an article that mentioned another teacher's use of death-related topics in creative writing exercises. Without any other preparation Ms. Cue assigned her students the task of writing their own obituaries. One result was a storm of protests from the parents to the principal about the bad dreams and other upsets some of the students were experiencing.

In another example, Clergyperson Heavy attended a conference where someone mentioned that many support groups for bereaved spouses were in operation. Heavy, without any other preparation, started a support group for widows. By the second meeting it was clear to Heavy that one widow tended to dominate the small group; she wanted to talk about her loss and she was upsetting the others. The nervous Clergyperson Heavy asked her not to return because she was so hostile and she resisted everyone's suggestions to her. One result was that she refused to allow anyone, especially a group, to help her.

The two stars of these examples were educated in their respective fields and both attempted to be helpful via the vogue of today; but evidently they did not suspect that they were stepping out of bounds, that they did not know how to proceed or how their efforts might be received. Even more sadly, they did not know that they did not know.

The popular attitude in our society seems to be that anyone can teach, any teacher can teach almost anything, or any counselor, psychologist, or social worker can help just about anyone needing those services regardless of client need for service. Some professionals in these fields also seem to believe this. In practice, however, even the relative truth is eminently different. Death Education requires more than education or training in a field. There is a body of knowledge, there are sets of skills, and there are attitudes essential for high quality Death Education. This is a critical matter for Death Education and represents a crucial challenge to members of the community of thanatologists.

In all of Death Education the *what* has received more attention than any other facet. Time and space here allow only for a few examples. As Death Education was emerging, professional journals began publishing articles, and books began to appear. In the middle 1960s a few colleges and universities began offering courses for credit, a few hospitals and long-term care facilities began relevant training courses and programs, and Kastenbaum and Kalish, in

1966, co-edited a quarterly newsletter that became the journal *Omega* in 1970. In 1967, Kutscher led the establishing of the Foundation of Thanatology; in 1971 the Foundation began publishing the quarterly *Archives of the Foundation of Thanatology*.

Indeed, the 1970s saw an explosion of growth and development. A variety of clinicians, researchers, and educators in 1974 formed the International Work Group on Death, Dying, and Bereavement; one of their tasks was the development of standards of care of the dying. Levitan, a health educator, led a small group to establish, in 1976, a national organization, the Forum for Death Education and Counseling. The Forum held annual conferences, and, in 1977, the Forum began publishing the *Newsletter*. The Forum is now known as the Association for Death Education and Counseling, and the *Newsletter* is now the *Forum Newsletter*. Also in 1977, publication of the journal *Death Education: Pedagogy, Counseling, Care–An International Quarterly*, with Wass, a psychologist, as editor began. The journal is known as *Death Studies*. The 1977, Volume 1, Number 1 of *Death Studies* was a bountiful issue with articles from Corr, Kastenbaum, Levitan, Nash-Conners-Gemperle, O'Connell-Kopel-Paris-Giardin-Batsel, Pine, and Sharapan.

Exciting growth and development continued all through the 1980s. Films, slides, audiotapes, and videotapes abounded. Television programs and movies focused upon Death Education topics. National talk shows invited death educators as guests. National organizations were encouraging and sponsoring meetings, workshops, training sessions, e.g., the National Funeral Directors Association, the National Hospice Organization, the American Cancer Society. The Forum for Death Education and Counseling became the Association for Death Education and Counseling (ADEC) and began several activities to improve the education of its constituencies: professional development workshops, differing each year; establishment of the National Certification Review Board with certification procedures for death educators and for grief counselors; coordination of annual certification courses; adoption of a new Code of Ethics; establishment of a Curriculum Task Force for developing standards by which others may evaluate death education materials and programs in schools. Several independent organizations also emerged, each with an emphasis on some part of Death Education.

All of the excitement and enthusiasm characteristic of the 1980s revealed some issues which we might consider. For one example, for a number of reasons funding agencies and institutions have been rather slow in making funds available for worthwhile projects of research, of program and materials development, and of dissemination. One of the major reasons, of course, is too many in need competing for too few resources, an old story.

As another example, in New York City, a staffer surveyed a large number of teachers by asking them to list the ten most important topics the curriculum should address. No one mentioned topics of death and loss. Our death-denying society (Weisman, 1972) continues in large measure to avoid death-related issues. Earlier this author surveyed the curriculum directors of six of the largest public school systems in the U.S. Among other things, a goal was to find out who was providing what Death Education at which level. For the purposes here, the most striking information was that only one of these large systems had an identifiable program, K-12, developed by teams of district teachers and staff. In a few other districts one teacher, working independently, per district had developed one unit of study. Except in the one district Death Education had, at best, only token recognition. Further, a few respondents reported that they had experienced considerable resistance to sex education in their districts, and Death Education was in about the same boat.

Some voices of opposition remind us that there are people, generally characterized as Christian religious fundamentalists, who are opposed to parts of the curriculum generally offered in schools. They tell us, for example, they are anti-science, as the schools teach it, because much of what is being taught stands contrary to what their fundamentalism teaches; they believe their idea of creationism should replace the concept of evolution. Concepts of self-study and introspection often are offered in schools as humanistic education. The fundamentalists label this *secular humanism*, and to them secular humanism is a religion. They would prefer to have their religion taught in schools in place of humanistic ideas, i.e., what they label as secular humanism. They believe humanistic activity presents a barrier between the person and God; helping a widow to examine her feelings about her bereavement diverts her attention which properly belongs on God, not on herself. These are examples of views that can serve as motivators for death educators to continue examining the nature and role of Death Education.

Another part of the *what* question is what are we doing: Are we educating or are we training? A general understanding is that education draws and teaches from a broad base. Many would say that the liberal arts are the core of education; they provide general knowledge and develop general intellectual capacities. Training, by contrast, is much more narrow in that it develops skills. A death educator certainly needs both. There are, at least, three problems here. One arises when the death educator's education is not sufficiently broad; the second arises when the education does not include professional training (an appropriate narrowing of focus); the third arises when the death educator receives only training. The challenge is to resolve these problems adequately.

Certainly there are many in our death-denying society who resist the idea of Death Education because it is a topical area they would rather avoid or ignore. They offer a wide range of reasons for not stepping into this area, and for us not to engage in Death Education. Thus we face questions about *why* Death Education. The *why* has been articulated fairly well in hundreds of thoughtful, sobering anecdotal reports. One particularly should be noted. Warren, (1989) in Australia, is a clinical psychologist who has an interest in philosophy. His call is for us to devote more attention to developing a clearer philosophy of Death Education. He says that of the variety of philosophies available, probably that which comes to us by way of personal construct psychology is most promising. It may be. What is readily apparent, though, is that little effort among death educators is visibly directed toward developing a philosophy of Death Education. An articulated philosophy or set of philosophies could form a lodestone guiding the directions we pursue and thereby strengthening the foundations of Death Education.

An earlier part of this paper referred very briefly to a few of the people who pioneered the development of Death Education and thanatology. Then the issues of the what, how, and why of Death Education were discussed. The paper concludes with some brief comments on the *who* of Death Education. Currently there are two groups to whom we should attend: the credentialed and the non-credentialed. The credentialed include those who, by virtue of education and experience, have achieved certification or comparable recognition as educators; they have demonstrated their competence in providing education to others. The non-credentialed have neither the education nor the experience to qualify as educators. Some members of both groups could qualify as death educators and find meaningful places within thanatology.

Qualified educators could become death educators by acquiring additional, supervised education and experiences in Death Education. Persons not yet qualified educators could become death educators by completing courses in basic teaching and learning, plus acquiring additional, supervised education and experiences in Death Education. The Association for Death Education and Counseling has teams of thanatologists who develop and implement standards and processes for certification of death educators and for grief counselors. Certification is available to both at the Associate and at the Professional Levels through the ADEC National Certification Review Board.

Currently there exist Master's level thanatology programs at three institutions: (1) Brooklyn College, Department of Health Education (begun in 1984); (2) New York University, School of Education, Health, Nursing, & Arts Professions, Department of Applied Psychology's Programs in Counseling (begun in 1985); and (3) The University of Florida at Gainesville, Department of Psychology (begun in 1987). Mount Ida College in Newton Centre, Massachusetts, currently has an application pending approval by the Massachusetts Board of Regents of Higher Education to offer an interdisciplinary Baccalaureate program in Bereavement Education.

We need to keep an eye out for those non-certified, talented, creative people who have the art, the skill, the compassion, and the good sense so surely needed in Death Education. They should be encouraged to join us as death educators, to pursue their professional development. Certification is not necessarily the "be all and end all," but it is a part of professional development, and continuous professional development is essential for each of us. Finally, enhanced sharing of ideas and dialogues will continue to develop thanatology research, creativity, and service, and will help ensure the future of the thanatology movement.

REFERENCES

Bloom, B. (ed.). 1956. *Taxonomy of Educational Objectives, Handbook I: Cognitive Domain*. New York: David McKay Co.

Feifel, H. (ed.). 1959. *The Meaning of Death*. New York: McGraw-Hill.

Feifel, H. (ed.). 1977. *New Meanings of Death*. New York: McGraw-Hill.

Kastenbaum, R. and B. Kastenbaum. 1989. *The Encyclopedia of Death*. Phoenix: The Oryx Press.

Krathwohl, D., B. Bloom, and B. Masia. 1964. *Taxonomy of Educational Objectives, Handbook II: Affective Domain*. New York: David McKay Co.

Mager, R. 1962. *Preparing Instructional Objectives*. Palo Alto: Fearon Publishers.

Raphael, B. 1983. *The Anatomy of Bereavement*. New York: Basic Books.

Rogers, C. 1957. The necessary and sufficient conditions of therapeutic personality change. *Journal of Consulting Psychology*, 21:95-103.

Warren, W. 1989. *Death Education and Research: Critical Perspectives*. New York: The Haworth Press, Inc.

Weisman, A. 1972. *On Dying and Denying*. New York: Behavioral Publications.

White, E.B. 1952. *Charlotte's Web*. Illustrated by Garth Williams. New York: Harper & Row.

Disseminating Our Thanatology Knowledge

Hannelore Wass

INTRODUCTION

We can consider at least three questions about our thanatology knowledge as we evaluate our area and assess our needs. First, how much have we produced and what is its quality? Second, how well have we spread this knowledge among ourselves, the next generation of thanatologists, among our colleagues in the mainstream disciplines, and among the general public? Third, how well have we translated our knowledge into action and applied it in practice?

While this article will focus mainly on the subject of dissemination, the prior question to consider, or course, is whether or not we *have* knowledge and wisdom worthy of dissemination. This means considering the even more fundamental question, "What is our field?" There is by no means complete agreement on what constitutes the field of death and dying. Even among specialists we have differing opinions. Still, most of us probably agree with Kalish (1988) that the field encompasses three core areas, dying, death, and bereavement. Not coincidentally, one of the major thanatology organizations, the International Work Group on Death, Dying and Bereavement, reflects this definition.

Some specialists would add destructive behavior as a fourth core area. Destructive behavior against self and others, by individuals or groups, is one of the most troubling contemporary issues. It might be thought of as a preventable social disease. Except for suicide, it is, however, one of the least studied topics. That in itself should

---

Hannelore Wass, PhD, is Professor of Educational Psychology, University of Florida, Gainesville, FL.

startle us. For example, Stark (1991) notes that despite its enormous significance for health, professionals in the health fields have paid little attention to homicide. He suggests that existing theories and models of prevention are as inadequate as is the database. Clearly, there are problems in a system of homicide investigation in which a large percentage of murders are undetected or no suspects are identified (Toufexis, 1989). Is this apparent lack of attention or concern a reflection of society's attitude toward the value of life?

The issue of AIDS hovers over us as a black shadow. Is it an "area" waiting to be adopted by us? Do we consider it a legitimate aspect of our field? Or is it about disease, health, sex, and drugs?

For this discussion, Kalish's definition of the core concepts in the field as death, dying, and bereavement are adapted. Of these core areas, dying and bereavement can be viewed as essentially concerned with finite processes. In terms of scientific inquiry, they seem feasible and accessible, and we view them to be clearly in the domain of the social/behavioral sciences. The third focal area, death itself, its meanings and interpretations, our individual and cultural stances toward it, is more elusive. It concerns something more fundamental, a general condition, a state. Here we cross over into philosophy, ethics, faith. But it is part of the stuff of the death movement, its roots and reach. Certainly, the movement has emphasized the importance of acknowledging and accepting our mortality (Feifel, 1959). Without question, we have increased death awareness and sensitivity to the issues of death. But our relative progress in this arena is difficult to measure.

In the areas of dying and bereavement we can boast of results. We have made progress in understanding the processes of dying and grief and mourning, in identifying the needs of the dying and bereaved and their families, and in discovering ways we can support and care for them. We have, in fact, generated a considerable amount of data in these areas. Whether we can call it "a body" of knowledge is another question. How valid, reliable, and authoritative these data are, is also not so easy to determine. In a sense, most knowledge is tentative, true only until proven incorrect. And our faith in the validity and reliability of our findings improves every time they are confirmed in further study. So we progress not so much in quantum leaps from ignorance to knowledge, but more in degrees of confidence.

Critics have charged that our work is short on theory. We should take this criticism seriously. Much theory-building is needed. For example, bereavement is currently one of the most widely studied subjects in our field. Yet there is not work that integrates the research. One reason for this lack lies in the difficulty one has comparing the work. There are few explicit theoretical models and few common concepts and terms. If we in the field do not speak the same language, how are we to communicate to professionals in other areas or to the general public? Theoretical formulations and conceptual models that do exist need to be refined, expanded, and tested.

Most particularly, we need to frame our research questions in the broader contexts of the major disciplines of which they are a part. To illustrate, we have made significant progress in the study of death fears and anxieties especially in methodology, and most especially in the development of measurement instruments. However, few of these instruments are clearly founded in psychological theory. The notable exception is the *Threat Index*, a measure of death anxiety based on Kelly's theory of personal constructs (Neimeyer, 1988). In addition to theories of cognition and cognitive consistency, we might consider theories of self-actualization, self concept, or other self theories for developing hypotheses about fears of death. No empirical studies on death-related fears based on Erik Erikson's theory of psychosocial development through the life span are recalled. This theory could be used as a basis for developing research questions about change and stability, individual differences, age, social and situational influences, and other factors that may influence death-related fears and concerns. There are few longitudinal studies that examine attitudes toward death across the life span, *with* or *without* theoretical anchorage.

We need to expand our experimental populations to be better able to make generalizations. For instance, most of the studies on fears of death have been done with college students, most of them undergraduate psychology majors. How much confidence can we have in the findings? In the study of grief, we have just within the past decade or so expanded our populations of younger and middle-aged adults to include older persons and children. We also need to do more evaluation and programmatic research—both outcome and process-oriented—to gain a better sense of how effective we are in practice, in clinical interventions, and in our educational efforts.

COMMUNICATING IN THE PROFESSIONS

Despite these shortcomings, we have developed a base of knowledge upon which to build further study and which to use as a tentative guide for clinical and practical application (Feifel, 1990). How well are we disseminating this knowledge?

One aspect of communications concerns the population that is addressed. In broadest terms, we can identify two populations; the professionals and the general public. We can think of the professionals as comprising three groups: the death, dying, and bereavement specialists, the students to be the next generation of specialists, and our colleagues in the major disciplines. Another aspect concerns the forms and forums we use.

Publications

Our field has an extensive book market. We are very productive in spreading knowledge in this forum. Commercial publishers have "warmed up" considerably to the subject of death in the past two decades or so. With the increasing popularity of the personal computer and "user friendly" software, desktop publishing has added another layer of death-related materials. The topics that are treated reflect, in general, the concerns of the field. Some topics are clearly more popular than others. Grief seems to be such a subject. Many different aspects are treated. For example, there are books on grief counseling and therapy, anticipatory grief, parental grief, children's grief, disenfranchised grief, grief when a child was murdered, grief following sudden infant death, and neonatal grief.

Books in thanatology can be classified, essentially, into four categories: (1) scholarly accounts such as research and clinical reports; (2) efforts at integrating knowledge from various sources such as textbooks and books of readings; (3) practical guides and handbooks; and (4) personal accounts. In addition to the great variety in themes, there also is considerable variation with respect to quality, similar to other evolving fields. Our area particularly may be vulnerable to work that is not channelled through an established peer review process. Books may be the forum in which such checks are more easily avoided than in other forums. The subject of death is a little bit like the subject of teaching. Most people think they know about teaching because they have personally experienced it. Some people consider themselves experts on death because they have had experience with death. Some excellent volumes have been published that are based on such personal experiences and undoubtedly have had a profound influence. But experience alone does not make one an expert in a scientific field.

There is no question that many of the books are used as references by thanatologists. Apparently a number of them are used as major resources. One can determine this is true by looking at how frequently authors cite these books in their research reports and particularly by noting the ratio of such citations to those from the journal literature.

Because many books are written in nontechnical language and do not have the typical "baggage" of scholarly work, i.e., detailed documentation, referencing, and footnoting, these books may appeal to the general public as well. Often the authors explicitly state such dual objectives, and many of the books in the field have become bestsellers.

There will continue to be much activity in book publishing. Death is obviously a marketable subject. That itself is some measure of the success as a movement. Because this is an evolving field, these books have a relatively short life span. We need continued scholarship and writing. Only a few titles tend to become classics; most of them become merely dated.

Journals are another major forum for professional communications. We have several journals that are specifically designed to publish thanatological knowledge. They include *Omega*, *Death Studies*, *The Hospice Journal*, *The Journal of Palliative Care*, *Loss, Grief and Care*, among others, and the most recently established journal, *Illness, Crises and Loss*. These journals are providing an important service in the field by permitting thanatologists to bring their work to their colleagues expeditiously. The specialty journals will continue to be a prominent part of the communication network. At the same time, however, it is important to have our work published in the journals of the major disciplines as well. In recent years editors of some major professions have been more inclined to publish papers dealing with death-related concerns. This is a promising development and will help to achieve needed integration of thanatology into its various parent disciplines.

There also is a surprisingly large market of audiovisuals that we can view as significant sources of knowledge. By now there are probably well over 1000 films, videotapes, or audiotapes available through commercial distributors or universities and health centers. It is well for us to examine these audiovisuals in terms of the quality of the knowledge they contain, because they are used in preparation and training.

Training and Preparation

Overall, we have made good progress in the arena of publications. But gaps remain. One important gap concerns the training of future generations of death, dying, and bereavement specialists. We have largely failed in this area. How many colleges and other professional schools offer ongoing programs in thanatology such as cognates, minors, or other academic tracks and practical, clinical training components? Currently, there are less than a handful of such programs at the university level in accredited institutions. (There may be more thanatology programs offered by external universities and correspondence schools.) Without systematic approaches to professional training, we will have difficulty establishing ourselves as a respected field. The conferences, summer institutes, seminars, workshops, and pre-conference courses that are presented by the organizations and agencies may be excellent. They are certainly an improvement over no training at all. But they are no substitute for established programs and curricula offered by the educational institutions.

Because our area is so new and we have not yet a tradition, and because the knowledge is fairly fluid and its quality variable, it is even more important that we provide structure, focus, continuity, and appropriate settings for our students.

We need to do what gerontology has done. Gerontology is useful as an example in several ways. Interest in the study of aging began approximately at the same time that interest in thanatology began (in the early 1950s). Unlike thanatology, however, it was boosted tremendously by federal and state legislation and, equally importantly, by the allocation of monies. Through the Older Americans Act, passed in 1964 and periodically amended and expanded, funds became available for research, program development, and training in the early 1970s. Today gerontology is an accepted and respected field of specialization. Most major universities and many smaller colleges have established academic programs in the area. Congress is not likely to pass legislation to assist our field (no "Death and Dying Act" for us). The fundraising efforts of organizations like the Foundation of Thanatology, therefore, are essential and can serve as a model for other organizations in the field.

The requisite for establishing programs for professional training is that we become fully accepted as a field or sector in the social/behavioral sciences, and in the health and other helping professions. An essential avenue for such acceptance is the incorporation of our knowledge into the major disciplines.

Mainstreaming

One approach to such integration, as mentioned, is for thanatology researchers to conceptualize their questions in multi-disciplinary terms, to anchor them in the broader context; in essence, to mainstream the problems. Another is to publish our work in the mainstream journals. A third is to communicate our knowledge at conferences and in written documents through the various organizations of the major disciplines.

GENERAL CURRICULA

Meanwhile, an important long-term way to facilitate the process of incorporation is to get the basics of our knowledge included in the curricula of the major disciplines. It is all well and good for us to offer the "death and dying" courses at our colleges and universities, but in most instances these courses are not part of required professional curricula. It is unrealistic to expect that every nursing, medical, and social work student, every student in psychology or sociology will take the death and dying courses that are offered. A more practical, if more difficult, approach is to present thanatological knowledge as integral components of standard courses and sequences of studies in the major disciplines.

To illustrate, during the Civil Rights Movement in the late 1960s and early 1970s, a new awareness and pride in one's ethnicity developed and black studies emerged on many college campuses and in high schools. Scholars had poured over archival records and identified contributions in literature, history, and sciences made by blacks. This material was then packaged into a course and introduced into various curricula as a special offering. The problem was that few students other than Afro-Americans enrolled in these courses. The knowledge reached only a fraction of the population for whom it was intended. It does not make good sense at that educational level to teach black history, white history, Spanish-American history, black or white literature, and so on. You teach American history, American literature. Since then, much progress has been made incorporating Afro-American contributions into the appropriate course syllabi. That is what is needed in the area of death and dying.

It is necessary to emphasize that the basic knowledge that has been developed in the past 40 years or so has not been incorporated into the professional curricula of the mainstream disciplines and fields in the behavioral/social sciences, nor in the various branches of the helping professions. There is little by way of sophisticated, state-of-the-art thanatological information and thinking contained in the professional curricula in medicine, nursing, social work, counseling, consulting or clinical psychology, psychiatry, or education. To this author's knowledge, there are no licensing or board examinations in these professions that include questions having to do with dying, death, or bereavement.

Textbooks

Textbooks are, of course, closely related to the general professional curricula. Death-related content similarly is absent in the standard texts of the various disciplines and fields in the behavioral and social sciences and the helping professions.

Such content is absent even in specialty texts in which it seems central and consequential. Consider gerontology texts. By definition, old people are survivors. They experience losses of significant persons in their lives including spouses, other relatives, friends, sometimes even children and grandchildren. In the gerontology texts are found extensive descriptions of the various losses old people experience as they age, such as sensory losses, losses in memory, motor acuity, stamina, health, and social roles. But human losses are strangely absent. Yet, we have gained much insight into the dynamics of grief, and in the recent past, have generated considerable knowledge specifically about grief in the elderly as well (Lund, 1989). There are a few notable exceptions, but even here, the content presented often is superficial and dated.

The question is how do we go about achieving such integration? It will take considerable brainstorming to answer it, and time commitment to do it, but it can be done.

OTHER AVENUES

Publishing some of our work in the established journals of our major disciplines significantly can assist in the process of disciplinary integration. This sort of linking should be happening at a faster rate than currently is the case.

Breakthroughs have not occurred yet in the journals of various branches of psychology, or education, nor in many journals in the health fields. Even when we submit our work to the mainstream journals, it may not be accepted. Editors may not view death as a significant or legitimate topic for their area or of little interest to their readers. Editors may have a personal aversion to the subject. One observation is that journals in the major fields sometimes publish material that is rather unsophisticated and does not present new information (although it may be new to the reviewers). One way to solve this problem is for thanatologists to volunteer to serve on the editorial boards of these journals.

Our own organizations can do a number of things that may assist in mainstreaming our knowledge. We could establish formal and information communications and dialogue among ourselves and the organizations of the major disciplines. We could establish structures and mechanisms among our own organizations that would facilitate collaboration and pursual of common objectives. We could form interest groups or even establish sections in death, dying, and bereavement within our various major disciplinary organizations. We could collaborate on the planning and presentation of symposia, panel discussions, or roundtables at regional and national meetings. Our organizations could develop and disseminate position papers and prepare various documents such as the International Work Group on Death, Dying, and Bereavement has been doing. There are numerous possibilities for communicating our knowledge to the professions.

PUBLIC EDUCATION

Perhaps the most challenging task of mainstreaming is to disseminate our knowledge among the public at large. Of course, public education is going on in various forms and forums, through books, pamphlets, the national press, the electronic media, through seminars, workshops, conferences, and other communications by word of mouth. But this kind of dissemination is neither systematic nor comprehensive.

One long-term and systematic approach to transmitting basic knowledge and wisdom about death, dying, and bereavement to the general public is through the mechanisms and processes of our public schools. There are at least four reasons why this is so.

First, transmitting the knowledge, skills, and practices of our society to our young is the primary role of the schools. Basic knowledge about death, dying, and bereavement is part of this culture and should be part of our young's cultural education. It should not be a political issue nor a matter of public debate. The scientific aspects of death are legitimate subject matter for education in the schools. They do not threaten the separation of church and state or interfere with parents' roles and rights, although schools need to take care to avoid dealing with issues of faith and personal convictions.

Second, the sort of integration suggested for the professional disciplines is best begun at the lower educational levels in order to provide the broadest possible foundation. In this approach, death and dying content is incorporated into various subjects in which it naturally fits. For example, in biology or the life sciences, teachers discuss the human life cycle in addition to that of plants and animals. In social studies, family planning, psychology or similar studies, teachers can teach about causes of death, about how people respond to death and loss, and basic skills in how they can help one another in times of crisis. In health classes, they can discuss life-threatening diseases, AIDS, destructive behaviors, healthy habits, and life styles. The key is that basic information is provided in several subject matters, at different times, different educational levels, in developmentally appropriate ways in the larger contexts, in a planned, structured, and coordinated fashion. When thanatological content is made part of the schools' regular curricular offerings in this way, it does not depend on individual initiative nor is it subject to political pressure.

Such long-term preventive and preparatory education is largely absent in our schools. A recent national survey found that fewer than a fifth of the middle and high schools, and only one in ten elementary schools, offer such education (Wass, Miller, and Thornton, 1990 a).

Third, integrating death and dying material naturally into the schools' curricula makes it more manageable. Because such education is foresighted rather than crisis-oriented, i.e., long-term rather than for the immediate situation, it is less likely to be stressful and emotionally taxing and more likely to be low-keyed. And because of these factors, teachers, administrators, and parents may find it easier to accept.

This kind of long-term systematic approach to death education should not replace crisis intervention programs in the schools. In fact, it may enhance them. Recent developments in school-based suicide intervention are encouraging. Also, leaders in this area are working to expand these programs to include prevention as well as intervention and post-vention.

Unfortunately many people who make decisions about public education remain unconvinced about the need for such death education for children. An enormous task of persuasion lies ahead. But, with recent developments in AIDS education, we have a dramatic example which shows that once there is a general perception of need, many groups and agencies, including parents, can effectively collaborate in introducing certain content into the schools' curricula (Wass, Miller, and Thornton, 1990 b). Health professionals, especially the thanatologists among them, are in an excellent position to influence public opinion in this respect simply by coming out in support of death education in the schools. In addition, they can lead such efforts in their own communities. In this way they can contribute substantially to the dissemination of basic thanatological knowledge.

Finally, there is an urgent need to teach young people appropriate attitudes and orientations toward death *as an antidote* to the kind of death education they are receiving through the popular culture of film, video, and music. There is a danger of a blurring of the distinction between education and entertainment. That should be of deep concern to thanatologists and educators. Death is grossly distorted in the popular culture, and violent death predominates. Perhaps what we need is a refiring of the death movement. It seems that in lifting the taboo of death, we may unwittingly have contributed to the current preoccupation and fascination, but with the kind of death that cries in the face of our ideals of humanity. What are we to make of this new license for death? Is it an index of some deep anxieties in the Zeitgeist? Or does it merely demonstrate the brilliant marketing psychology of the entertainment industry?

Regardless of how we answer the question, we should be impressed by the power of popular culture for shaping thinking, perceptions, attitudes, and ultimately, behavior. We already have evidence or good reason to suspect that filmed aggression increases aggressive behavior in young viewers and that constant bombardment and exposure to violence leads to apathy. What consistently is presented without critical comment can be understood as the standard or norm. Children, and adults as well, overestimate the incidence of violence and homicide in their communities and in the country. There is little portrayal of the pain and suffering associated with death, and what little is shown, often is shallow.

Few people die naturally in film, TV, or on video. Today personal experience with natural death is uncommon in childhood. How do children learn about grief? Where do they learn empathy and caring for others? Should we not be concerned that we teach young people about the value and preciousness of life? Should they not learn to be enraged and ready to act against those who commit atrocities against others? And should we not be concerned that we instill a desire to improve the quality of life for all and to preserve the earth?

Perhaps it is a good time to redefine our field, our objectives, our commonalities and divergencies, and, perhaps, our mission. This will enhance our ability to develop, disseminate, and use new thanatology knowledge, wisdom, and skills.

REFERENCES

Feifel, H. (ed.). 1959. *The Meaning of Death*. New York: McGraw-Hill.

Feifel, H. 1990. Psychology and death: Meaningful rediscovery. *American Psychologist*. 45(4):537-543.

Kalish, R.A. 1988. The study of death: A psychosocial perspective. In H. Wass, R.A. Neimeyer, and F.M. Berardo (eds.), *Dying: Facing the Facts. Second Edition*. Washington, DC: Hemisphere Publishing Corporation, 55-75.

Lund, D.A. (ed.) 1989. *Older Bereaved Spouses: Research with Practical Applications*. New York: Hemisphere Publishing Corporation.

Neimeyer, R.A. 1988. Death anxiety. In H. Wass, R.A. Neimeyer, and F.M. Berardo (eds.), *Dying: Facing the Facts. Second Edition*. Washington, DC: Hemisphere Publishing Corporation, 97-136.

Stark, E. 1991. Preventing primary homicide: A reconceptualization. In D. Leviton (ed.), *Horrendous Death, Health, and Well-Being*. New York: Hemisphere Publishing Corporation, 109-136.

Toufexis, A. 1989. Coroners who miss all the clues. *Time*, August 14, 61.

Wass, H., M.D. Miller and G. Thornton. 1990 a. Death education and grief/suicide intervention in the public schools. *Death Studies*. 14(3);253-268.

Wass, H., M.D. Miller, and G. Thornton. 1990 b. AIDS education in the U.S. public schools. *AIDS Education and Prevention*, 2:213-219.

Individual Rights vs. State Interests: Ethical Concerns in Thanatology

T. Patrick Hill

One of the phrases that has dogged the so-called right-to-die debate almost from inception is "the slippery slope." Constantly on the lips of those who claim to be pro-life, the phrase has been used to warn against stepping on to a sliding moral landscape in which human life becomes all too expendable. Typically, it is heard in those cases where a patient has been diagnosed, for example, as in a persistent vegetative state. Although the prognosis is hopeless, it is not terminal. As a result, the patient can be kept alive as long as medical treatments, like artificial feeding, are provided. Clearly, patients in this condition, even those who have executed in advance medical directives, must be handled with extreme care because they are vulnerable. And because they are so vulnerable, any decisions that are made to withhold or stop treatment can be viewed, so the slippery slope argument goes, as setting a precedent for decisions about treating other vulnerable groups, such as the severely mentally retarded. If today we can find it within ourselves to approve not treating a patient in a persistent vegetative state, then tomorrow we will find it that much easier not to treat, for example, someone diagnosed with quadriplegia.

Apart from a severe weakness in the logic of this argument, there is scant empirical evidence in current medical practice to suggest that decisions to stop treatment taken in cases of patients diagnosed with one illness have become the precedent for decisions regarding patients with another illness. There is even less evidence that, as a

---

T. Patrick Hill, is Director of Education, CHOICE in DYING, New York, NY.

society, we have become psychologically tolerant of stopping life-sustaining medical treatments in general because of an accumulation of particular cases like that of Karen Ann Quinlan, where decisions to stop treatment have been made.

This is not to say that we are not growing more tolerant of stopping medical treatments, the direct result of which is death. But the source of this tolerance is, paradoxically, a growing awareness of the capacity of technological medicine to maintain biological life even in the absence of sapient life, coupled with profound doubts about the desirability of using such capacity routinely. It seems reasonable then to say that the slippery slope argument, presented as it usually is, is logically suspect and factually erroneous. Despite that, the slippery slope argument can be posed in the same medical context. To be of use, however, it has to be couched in different terms.

Where decisions have been made to withhold or stop medical treatment, in addition to medical grounds, they have been justified legally and ethically on the basis of the autonomy of the individual. The critical question to which this gives rise is whether, by accepting the legitimacy of individual autonomy, we are undermining societal interests in protecting the inviolability of human life? Whether, in other words, we are putting individual rights on an unavoidable collision course with non-negotiable community interests? Couched in this fashion, the slippery slope argument becomes credible in relation to logic and fact. There is a direct relationship between the individual acting as an individual and the individual acting as a constituent of the larger human community. The individual, paradoxically, is defined in large measure in relation to the community. For its part, the human community is, again paradoxically, nonexistent in the absence of autonomous individuals. The two, in fact, only exist by means of a creative tension between two forces: the centripetal force by which the individual seeks out a larger center of existence, namely, the human community; and the centrifugal force which allows the individual to escape the anonymity latent in any communal existence. In this paradigm, there are two constants – the individual and the community. The major variables are the two forces and the dynamics involved in either seeking or avoiding the center. If a slippery slope exists at all, it will be found here where decisions to withhold or stop medical treatment, justified on the basis of individual autonomy, may entail negative consequences for the substantial interests of the human community at large.

Using this paradigm to frame the issue of a slippery slope, we can, by means of select case studies, determine empirically how it might manifest itself, and how seriously it has to be taken. Two that immediately present themselves as appropriate for this analysis are those of Karen Ann Quinlan and Nancy Cruzan. Both have been settled in court and represent two decisions which are precedent-setting but for very different reasons. Despite their differences, the two cases illustrate the way individuals can, in the exercise of their autonomy, appear to challenge interests the human community has in protecting the inviolability of human life.

The remarkable thing about the case of Karen Ann Quinlan is that, since 1976 when it was decided, its public policy significance has begun to outstrip its legal significance. While the case was before the New Jersey courts, it had already begun to give form and substance to the possibility of real conflict between the rights of individuals to control the circumstances of their death and society's interests in protecting the inviolability of human life. Whatever the legal outcome at that time, it was clear that more was on trial than legal matters narrowly defined.

None recognized this perhaps as clearly as the justices of the New Jersey Supreme Court. Sensing what was at stake not only for Karen Quinlan herself, but also for society, should the request of Quinlan's parents to withdraw treatment from their daughter be granted, they created a formula which was designed to balance the claims of personal autonomy with the community's sense of its collective security. It is clear from the words of the formula that the mutual claims of individual and community have legal standing. When they conflict, as they threatened to in Quinlan, there has to be a way of establishing whether the claims of the individual or the community have priority. And when a priority is established, it remains to devise a way to grant the claims of one party, in this case Quinlan, without fundamentally compromising the claims of the other party, namely the community in this case. In other words, advancing the interests of one party without, by doing that, approaching what could become a slippery slope for the other party.

How the members of the New Jersey Supreme Court weighed the nature of Quinlan's claims to determine the circumstances of her death and the implications of those claims for the community can be seen in the following remarkable words. "We think that the state's interest (in the preservation of life) weakens, and the individual's right to privacy grows as the degree of bodily invasion (life-sustaining medical procedures) increases and the prognosis dims. Ultimately, there comes a point at which the individual's right overcomes the state's interest."[1] By virtue of this statement, the court did two critical things here. It asserted that Karen Quinlan had a constitutionally protected right to privacy and ruled that the "termination of treatment pursuant to the right of privacy is, within the limitations of this case, ipso facto, lawful."[2] Any counter claims by the state, would, as a consequence, be unjustified.

It is clear from a careful reading of its proceedings that the New Jersey Supreme Court did not view itself as setting a precedent on behalf of Karen Quinlan's specific interests that might subsequently work to the detriment of community interests. On the contrary, the court recognized that Quinlan's medical condition and the implications of continuing treatment in her condition presented society with an unprecedented constitutional challenge. By virtue of the medical technology being used to maintain Quinlan's life, the state could press its interests in protecting human life to an unprecedented degree. To make sure that that unprecedented degree did not become an unwarranted degree, the court declared that a constitutionally protected right of individual privacy could be invoked.

In this way, the New Jersey Supreme Court reinterpreted the relationship between the individual and society so as to reflect the realities of current medical capabilities. By doing this, the court also guaranteed the continuation of the tension essential to healthy relations between the individual and his community. Finally, the court's reinterpretation was phrased in a way that provided the means to determine the circumstances of death where the preferences of the individual conflict with those of society.

In many respects, the case of Nancy Cruzan, who resided in Missouri, is similar to Karen Quinlan's. Both women had suffered neocortical damage that left them in a persistent vegetative state. But unlike Quinlan, Cruzan was kept alive by means of artificial nutrition and hydration supplied through tubes inserted in her stomach. The continuation of treatment for Cruzan offered little beyond maintaining a medically futile situation. As a result, her parents requested permission to stop treatment so that Nancy Cruzan might be allowed to die.

When the Missouri State Supreme Court addressed the case, it clearly recognized the possibility of conflict between individual autonomy and society's collective interests posed by the request of Cruzan's parents. Since the case before it was so similar to the Quinlan case, the Missouri court could, presumably have adopted the substance of the legal argument advanced by its sister court, applying them as needed to Cruzan. That after all is what many other courts had done since 1976, convinced, apparently of the essential correctness of the Quinlan decision. Not only did the Missouri court not find for Cruzan, it also rejected the constitutional grounds on which the New Jersey court had based its decision in favor of Quinlan. In doing what it did, the Missouri Supreme Court advanced a radically different understanding of the relationship between the individual and his society, in the apparent belief that in that relationship the only force that existed is the centripetal force. To view the relationship otherwise, particularly where an individual wished to determine the circumstances of his death, was to threaten the interests of the state. Here indeed was a slippery slope at the bottom of which would be found the destruction of the collective interests of society.

To avoid it, the Missouri court embraced what might be called an ideological vitalism, or a presumption favoring the value of biological life as something overriding any other value. On the basis of such a presumption, any interest in the preservation of human life would have to be considered extremely strong. It is not surprising therefore that when the Missouri court applied the presumption to the Cruzan case it declared that the state's interests in the preservation of human life are absolute. As the court expressed it, "The state's interest in life embraces two separate concerns: an interest in the prolongation of the life of the individual patient and an interest in the sanctity of life itself."[3] The court may declare these interests to be separate, but it is perfectly clear that the first interest derives directly from the second. Again, to use the court's own words:

"Given the fact that Nancy is alive and the burdens of her treatment are not excessive for her, we do not believe her right to refuse treatment, whether that right proceeds from a constitutional right to privacy or a common law right to refuse treatment, outweighs the immense, clear fact of life in which the state maintains a vital interest."[4] But given the fact that you and I are alive and the burdens of future medical treatment will not be excessive for us, would this court also believe that our right to refuse treatment outweighs the immense, clear fact of life in which the state maintains a vital interest? If the court says yes, and logically there is nothing to prevent it from doing so, then we may be looking at a sleeping slippery slope of totalitarian proportions. In other words, the premise is that individual rights are subordinate to state's interests. In logic at least there is a correlation between the value placed in something and the lengths one might go to protect the object of value. But there is good logic and there is bad logic, with the latter known usually by its faulty premises or conclusions or both.

In this case, the premise is suspect because it poses serious challenges to the individual as a moral agent and the subject of legal rights. That, in turn, poses equally serious consequences for society which functions best when the individuals comprising it function as moral agents and the subject of legal rights. But by accepting the presumption favoring the most elemental level of human life at any cost, the Missouri court was prepared, it seems, to supercede the moral standing of individuals and deprive them of fundamental rights. Among those rights are the common law and constitutional rights of equal protection, privacy and liberty. The court may have been persuaded that the only way to secure the collective interests of society was to keep Nancy Cruzan alive, despite her extreme medical condition, in the belief that a central interest of society is the inviolability of human life. But in light of the serious consequences of this persuasion to both society and individual, one has to ask whether it is justified, or indeed necessary?

Faced with the same dilemma in Quinlan, the New Jersey Supreme Court, while it accepted the principle of the inviolability of human life as a legitimate state interest, thought otherwise.[5] At bottom, the reason for the difference seems to lie in the fact that the New Jersey court focused on the medical plight of the patient. In this vein, the court declared, "We glean from the record here that physicians distinguish between curing the ill and comforting and easing the dying; that they refuse to treat the curable as if they were dying, or ought to die, and that they have sometimes refused to treat the hopeless and dying as if they were curable."[6] Alluding to expert testimony it had heard, the court went on to add that many physicians have refused to inflict an undesired prolongation of the process of dying on a patient in an irreversible condition when it is clear that such "therapy" offers neither human nor humane benefit.[7] Accordingly, the court concluded, "We think these attitudes represent a balanced implementation of a profoundly realistic perspective on the meaning of life and death and that they respect the whole Judeo-Christian tradition of regard for human life."[8] Significantly, it was the opinion of this court that just as these attitudes were consistent "with the moral matrix of medicine, 'to heal,' very much in the sense of the endless mission of the law, 'to do justice.'"[9]

The phrase, 'to do justice' is very much to the point in the present discussion, where the rights of the individual appear to be pitted against the interests of society, and where the court is attempting to strike a balance between conflicting claims. But as the New Jersey court was acutely aware, this balance "is particularly difficult to perceive and apply in the context of the development by advanced technology of sophisticated and artificial life-sustaining devices."[10] In the absence of a discriminating sense of the reasonable use of such life-sustaining devices with patients like Quinlan or Cruzan, there is the possibility of what the New Jersey court called the forced sustaining of an irreversibly doomed patient.[11] The operative word is forced and implies the possibility of the violation of the rights of an individual, even though, in this case, the individual happens to be a grossly incompetent patient.

Because of its focus on the plight of the patient and the protection of Quinlan's rights, the New Jersey court argued on the assumption that incompetence does not compromise either those rights or their exercise. The locus of those rights continues to be the individual, as distinct from her society, and therefore those rights are exercised primarily in the individual's best interests. The Missouri court proceeded in marked contrast. Largely because of its focus on an ideology of vitalism, it argued on the assumption that whatever rights an incompetent patient had, given her condition of incompetence, those rights were best subsumed under the aegis of state's interests. Whereas the New Jersey court assumed that the most effective defense of incompetent patients against possible abuse is the defense of their continuing to exercise their common law and constitutional rights, the Missouri court argued that the defense of state's interests in the protection of life offered the best defense of individual rights. It saw no need, as a result, to allow Cruzan's family to decide, by way of a substituted judgment, whether treatment could or should be continued. Unlike the New Jersey court, the Missouri court seemed oblivious to the implications of medical technology and discounted the threat it represented of forcing the prolongation of the process of dying. As a result, it failed to appreciate the risk of advancing state's interests at an unwarranted cost to individual rights. In rejecting the principle of substituted judgment, the Missouri court only served to increase that risk.

It is obvious that court cases, by definition, create winners and losers. That is true in the case of Nancy Cruzan and the case of Karen Ann Quinlan. In formulating its decision, the New Jersey Supreme Court weighed in the balance individual rights and state's interests and allowed individual rights to take precedence over state's interests within the limitations of Quinlan's case. In so doing, it was able to calculate up to what point individual rights could be exercised without jeopardizing legitimate and essential state's interests, such as the collective interest in the protection of human life. Within that calculus we are all winners—individuals and society. The Missouri court failed to see the need for balance as it addressed the conflicting claims of individual autonomy and societal collective interests embodied in the plight of Nancy Cruzan. As a result, it failed to determine acceptable levels of loss and gain above and below which it could not go without allowing an essentially unjust situation to emerge. A situation, that is, in which the condition of protecting one party's interests is the deprivation of another party's rights. Under that condition, we are all losers. Left unrecognized for what it really is, ideological vitalism has all the makings of a real slippery slope.

NOTES

1. In re Quinlan, 70 N.J. 10, 355 A.2d 647, cert. denied sub nom. Garger v. New Jersey, 429 U.S. 922 (1976), overruled in part, In re Conroy, 98 N.J. 321, 486 A. 2d 1209 (1985)
2. In re Quinlan, supra, 70 N.J. 10, 355 A.2d at 53
3. Cruzan v. Harmon, 760 SW2d 408 (Mo 1988), cert granted, 106L. Ed. 2d 587 (1989) at 419
4. Cruzan v. Harmon, supra, 760 SW2d at 424
5. In re Quinlan, supra, 70 N.J. 10 A.2d at 4
6. In re Quinlan, supra, 70 N.J. 10 A.2d at 47
7. In re Quinlan, supra, 70 N.J. 10 A.2d at 47
8. In re Quinlan, supra, 70 N.J. 10 A.2d at 47
9. In re Quinlan, supra, 70 N.J. 10 A.2d at 47
10. In re Quinlan, supra, 70 N.J. 10 A.2d at 47
11. In re Quinlan, supra, 70 N.J. 10 A.2d at 48

Children and Death: Directions for the 90s

Myra Bluebond-Langner

What problems should thanatologists address in the next decade? More specifically, how should thanatologists interested in the care and treatment of terminally ill children proceed? Let us take our direction from the children.

Our first speaker is a sixteen-year-old boy diagnosed two years prior with lymphoma:

> Their relapses worry me sometimes because they thought that someday they'd be sure and they could go on with their lives and it didn't turn out that way. So, once in a while I think maybe I will relapse and I won't be around very long. It makes me wonder whether I should just give up chemotherapy altogether and just live my life the best I can for a couple of months of whatever. Or just go out and have a good time because you really don't know what the future holds.

What does one say to such a child? How should one respond? In the future, as in the past, we will be searching for what to say to children with life-threatening illnesses. I use the word "searching" because I believe that we can never finally conclude that we understand the dying child's world and move on to other questions. Changes in both medicine and society require that we constantly evaluate our precepts about talking to dying children. It is only when we understand what children know about their diseases, what

---

Myra Bluebond-Langner, PhD, is Professor of Anthropology, Rutgers University, Camden, NJ.

their world is like, and how they communicate that we have the tools for such a task.

For example, in the above quotation we see that this dying child knows of peers who are not doing as well as peers who are cured. Indeed sixty percent of all children diagnosed with childhood cancer will survive. In the year 2000, 1 out of every 1000 nineteen-year-olds will be a survivors of childhood cancer.

For a long period of time, during the first years of treatment, children from both groups have a great deal of contact with each other—in waiting rooms, treatment centers, hospital floors and camps for children with cancer. What is it like for the child who will not survive to be around those who will?

Another consequences of the increased longevity of childhood cancer patients is the increased number of survivors is that they now compose an adolescent peer group. The bonds that form are significant and strong. In a study of children who attend cancer camp it was found that in addition to the contact that office visits and hospitalizations afford, over half the attendees of such camps remain in contact via letters, phone calls and informal visits (Bluebond-Langner, Perkel, and Goertzel, 1990; 1991). Contact was not related to age, diagnosis or state of health, but rather to feelings of comraderie, acceptance, understanding and support.

The children's relationship with other children with cancer were, however, not a substitute for relationships with healthy peers. These relationships were deeply prized, but difficult to maintain. The patient's relations with well peers is an important area for study. We need to know more about the world the child with cancer reenters. For example, we need to know how healthy children view children with cancer. What do they see as their strengths and weaknesses? What do they expect from them? What sorts of activities are they willing to engage in with them socially? This information is essential if we are to help the child negotiate the complex social relationships that follow on a new identity, different from the one the child had before he or she became ill.

We also need to be mindful of the impact of social changes and scientific advances on adults in the dying child's world—the physicians and the parents. Both are entrusted, in different ways and to different degrees, with the well being of the ill child. The death of a child represents failure to one in such a role. Fifteen years ago, the success of a treatment was measured by the number of months it extended the patient's life. Survival was the exception, not the rule. Today, as noted before, that situation has changed, and no doubt, survival rates will continue to improve in the next decade.

One wonders, however, if this success does not make the death of a child in a way harder—harder because it is less frequent, because it comes in the midst of tremendous advancements in care and treatment. As recently as fifteen to twenty years ago, one could say that the death of a child from cancer was difficult for physicians because it evidenced their almost total impotence in the face of the disease. Today, what does a child's death from cancer mean? Is it felt all the more keenly because many children do survive? Does it arouse feelings of self doubt or guilt—"Did I do everything possible for this child? If I can cure others, why did this child die?"

We cannot assume that fewer deaths and progress in the treatment of childhood cancer make it easier for caregivers. The impact of medical progress on physicians' responses to death is something which requires constant examination. The results of such a study must, of course, be used to reassess the information and education presented to physicians so that they will be able to respond to their terminally ill patients.

Changes in societal attitudes can alter the behavior of the other significant adults in the dying child's world—that of his or her parents. In the early 70s for example, there was little for parents to do in the face of a disease such as cancer. The result of their most diligent efforts was, like that of the physicians, something to be measured in increased months of life. They could not provide much beyond creature comforts. Sometimes they would try to protect their children from awareness of their fatal prognosis.

Parents today are less passive than they were ten and twenty years ago. They are less yielding to the demands of institutions such as hospitals and less cowed by authority figures such as physicians. Parents are more demanding, more likely to look for alternatives—second opinions, even radically alternative modes of care. Protecting one's child has assumed a more active character, one of advocacy.

Parents also are more willing to be open with their children when given appropriate support. The differences in parental approaches to health care professionals and to communication with their children has important implications for our work.

It should be clear that work in one of the first areas that thanatologists addressed—what do ill children know of death and how should we talk with them about it—can never be exhausted. Research must be ongoing and the results must be used to prepare caregivers anew for dealing with a terminally ill patient.

For further directions in thanatological research let us listen to the words of a fifteen-year-old girl with cystic fibrosis, moderate disease.

> I was shocked when Toby died. I knew she was sick in the last few years, but, still, Toby was so much older than the rest of us.
>
> Sharon's sicker than I thought she was. She's having that operation. She's scared. She didn't want to talk about it. She always seemed so healthy to me because of her attitude. Her attitude hides a lot of it. But I listened to her for about five minutes and I realized how sick she was.
>
> Lucy's sick. Lucy's always sick.
>
> I didn't know Alice that well, but I was here (in the hospital) when she died. I was talking on the phone one day and I smiled and we had eye contact and the next night she died and I knew when she died. I just felt it. And I walked to my room and sat down. And the nurse came in five minutes later and she goes, "You know, don't you?" And I go, "Yeah. I felt it." There's like something, a part of you dies, each time a CF patient dies. It's like we're all part of one. We are. Especially when Toby died. I guess Bev and Toby.
>
> When I found out they died, they were the hardest. Bev because of her attitude. She was such a little spit. She was the funniest person. No way she's going to die. She was just too active. She's got too much of a will. No way. I knew she didn't do her treatments at home. And she really didn't take her pills or anything. She was so naughty. But she was a fighter.
>
> And so I thought "Oh, Bev will always make it. She'll pull

> through." (Starts sobbing.) She can't. Because if she goes that means I'm going to go. Because I'm not as strong as Bev was.

While childhood cancer remains a major cause of death in children, it is not the only one. Many children suffer from diseases which run a much longer course; indeed, they may not die from their "childhood illness" until they reach adulthood. It is important to understand these children—to understand what it is like to live for ten, even twenty years, with a disease which ultimately becomes terminal.

The study of children with cystic fibrosis (CF) and their families provides some direction for us. Cystic fibrosis is the most common, lethal, genetically-transmitted disease in the United States. There is, as yet, no reliable prenatal or carrier detection test. The median age of survival is 21 years. By the time a child with CF is 12 or 14 years old, he or she has known several other children who have had CF and died. What do you say to such a child when yet another peer dies?

What do you say to children who, while certainly not dying, not even near death, are frailer than other children, than many CF patients for that matter; who suffer from complications of progressive lung disease, regularly battle more intractable infections, struggle to keep weight on, try to breathe without coughing lest their friends become suspicious and start to ask questions that they don't want to answer, or worse yet, draw away?

How do you help these children plan realistically for the future, albeit a diminished one? What about dating, marriage, sterility in males, the dangers in childbearing for females? Successfully dealing with these issues in the 90s and into the next century, which the newly diagnosed children will see, requires understanding of how these patients and their families handle the disease now.

These families act to contain the intrusion the disease makes into their lives. They try to maintain some modicum of normalcy, some level of control for as long as possible. The strategies that they use to achieve a sense of normalcy and control in the face of this demanding and devastating illness have consequences for the care and treatment of these children and their families.

For example, in the first year following diagnosis after the routines for care are established and the family is assured that the patient is doing well, families try to distance themselves from CF. They try to avoid reminders of the disease and its consequences. It is not unusual for families at this point in the disease process to begin to miss office appointments, to cease participating in parent groups or fundraising activities, to refrain from talking about CF. As one father explained:

> When you talk about it, you think about it and I think that's when you start to center your life around it. I don't want to hide it because I know it's there and I accept it, but on the other hand I didn't want to build my life around it, and I don't want to build my kids' lives around it. I want them to lead as normal a life as possible.

The desire for a normal life is palpable, and if achievement of that sense of normalcy means altering the realm of normal to accommodate changes in the patient's condition, so be it. So parents and well siblings often will minimize the patient's condition, focus on aspects of the patient's condition that are not indicative of advancing lung disease, but could be had by children with less catastrophic diseases.

This is not to say that patients and their family members deny what is happening, but rather that they choose to compartmentalize information about the disease and the patient's condition. Family members sort through the information that they have about their illness in such a way that particular kinds of information can be kept from immediate awareness. Parents, patients and well siblings feel this is necessary "for one's own sanity," "to keep on going," "to get done what needs to be done," or "to get on with your life."

Getting things done and getting on with one's life may require not doing all the treatments the physicians require. As one mother explained:

> There is just so much to do. We just can't seem to do it all and have any kind of a normal life—so we skip some treatments. At least that way we do the others. Otherwise it's too much and we wind up doing nothing. And, anyway, I'm not sure the treatments do all that much.

This quote also speaks to the issue of compliance, or more commonly its reciprocal, non-compliance. Like the term denial, compliance is a judgmental term. It is part of a mind set that insidiously and, it could be argued, unnecessarily increases the tension that exists between parents and caregivers. We would do well to throw out notions of compliance, non-compliance and denial, not just because they create tension and make bad situations worse, but also because they do not advance our understanding of the problem or help us to meet our goals.

On the one hand, we tell families to get on with their lives, plan for the child's future, the child is doing well enough that attending to how he or she is doing in school should be a priority. Yet on the other hand, when we insist on a physical therapy regimen that uses two to three hours of every day, how can that parent or patient get on with the business of living? This is not to say that we should encourage families to abandon therapy, but rather we should help them to choose among alternatives so that they can fulfill the other part of the prescription—get on with their lives, plan, do, and live with CF.

Further directions for research in the field of children living with catastrophic illness are found in the following comments by two well siblings of children with cystic fibrosis:

> My mom always asks me how come I never go down to the hospital to see my sisters. (His two sisters who have CF.) I don't want to go to the hospital. I don't want to go down there and see them in the hospital. It's not the fact that I don't want to go see them. It's just that I know what's going to happen. You know it's inevitable. You know the progression of the disease will get worse. That's inevitable. I get worried when she gets sick. Like when she had chicken pox, I was really worried about her. And I was. I sort of prayed every night that, you know, nothing happened. I get worried. And she is just sort of there and you can tell that there is really something wrong.

For many years we have spoken of the need to look at the impact that chronic and terminal illnesses have on well siblings. We have acknowledged their neglected status in care and research. But what have we done? The literature on the impact of chronic and terminal illnesses on well siblings is in a sorry state. Review of the literature in the field reveals myriad contradictions. Articles claim that having a sibling with a chronic or terminal illness has a positive effect, has a negative effect, or has no significant or appreciable effect on the well siblings.

These contradictions reflect a lack of attention to (1) the ways in which well siblings views and behaviors vary over the course of the illness; and (2) the role that the patient's condition and the parents' responses to it play in the well siblings' views and behaviors.

The impact of having a sibling with a life-threatening illness varies over the course of the illness. The well siblings' views and responses are part of a complex process involving (1) the patient's condition and experiences with the illness; (2) the well siblings' assessment of the patient's condition and experiences; (3) the parents' responses to the care the disease requires and the concerns it engenders; and (4) the well siblings' interpretation of those responses.

For example, in the early periods of the illness when the patient is doing relatively well, without frequent exacerbations or hospitalizations, and therapy is limited to once, or at most, twice a day, the parents speak infrequently about the patient's condition, except perhaps to mention how well the patient is doing. They relate participation in numerous extracurricular activities and easy recoveries from minor colds and flus. Then the well sibling sees CF as a condition one does things for. In the words of one well brother:

> There's a lot she has to do for her CF. But it's like she doesn't have it, except for her therapy and all which she acts is like a normal routine. I mean most of the time I forget she has it cause things become quite routine. I just forget about it. I don't think about it a whole lot.

Like their parents, the well siblings call attention to just how much the patient is like other children who do not have CF. At this point in the illness the well sibling feels justified in making demands for attention, privileges, and special foods like the patient is getting. He or she makes demands openly and directly, and some even admonish parents for spoiling the patient.

As the patient's condition begins to deteriorate, when exacerbations and hospitalizations become more frequent, infections more difficult to treat, complications more apparent, and the demands for carefar more difficult to accommodate, parents focus more attention on the patient. Goals, plans, and hopes for the patient's future are severely reduced, and with them, a sense of normal life.

At this time well siblings are reluctant to voice their demands for attention directly. This does not mean that they do not make their needs known in other ways such as poor school performance and exaggerated weight gain.

Noting the changes in the patient's condition and the parents' responses to it, the well sibling comes to see CF as a chronic, progressive incurable disease that shortens the life span. As one well brother explained:

> But I still get worried about my sister. I just know that with CF you could die from it and you get all skinny and your lungs fill up with mucus and you can't breathe and you die.

Acknowledging a shortened life span or terminal prognosis for persons with CF does not necessarily mean acknowledging that one's own sibling will die at an early age from CF. While the well sibling may link incurable and terminal, they do not necessarily internalize death as an outcome for their own brother or sister, at least not in the near future.

There is an attempt to distance oneself and one's siblings from the imminence, if not eventuality, of death. Well siblings speak of other things that still can be done. They carefully note the differences between their sibling's experiences and those of other patients who have died. They sprinkle their remarks with conditions and qualifiers, for example, "Her chances are almost zero." Cystic fibrosis is a despised enemy to be fought. Many well siblings become more protective of the patient. They find it difficult not to worry.

It is important to point out, however, that once well siblings see CF as a progressive, incurable, life-threatening illness, they are reluctant to share their view with their parents and the patient. This reluctance is often with full recognition that the patient not only knows the prognosis, but also that people are not willing to talk about it. Significantly, if at this point siblings do not share information and distance is created in their relationship it can last until the patient's death.

With advances in CF care and research, patients and their families will be able to enjoy relatively normal lives for much longer periods of time. Even now, as in the case of other life-threatening diseases, it is not unusual to find well siblings growing up and leaving home before the disease begins to take its toll. For them, growing up with a brother or sister with a catastrophic illness will have a far different effect than it did/does on those who grew up with someone who became severely ill and died in their developmental years.

In summary, if we are to be successful in working with the families of chronically and terminally ill children, we will need to know how family members perceive the course of the disease – the natural history and the significant turning points in the illness. We also will need to understand how family members deal with the care the disease requires and the concerns it engenders. More specifically, we will need to be familiar with the ways in which family members (1) manage the tasks of care; (2) process the information that they receive about the patient's condition and the disease; (3) deal with reminders of the illness; (4) approach difference from others; (5) conceptualize time, the future; and (6) assess and set priorities in the family.

Finally, attention needs to be paid to the AIDS epidemic. It is clear that the impact of this disease on our society and its institutions will be devastating. No commentary on the direction of thanatology can ignore this disease.

Understanding the social worlds of children with AIDS is a formidable task. The disease differs from other life-threatening diseases from which children have suffered during the last thirty years, in at least four significant ways. First, AIDS is symbolically highly charged. No other disease produces such strong reactions, moral and otherwise. Second, the children have contracted the disease from a stigmatized population. Third, the parents of these children are often dying or dead. Fourth, the population from which these children come is, for the foreseeable future, poor, Black, and Hispanic.

Any measures we develop, any suggestions we offer for the care of these children must come from a thorough understanding of these children's experience, from knowledge of their social worlds. This is data we do not have, and which would be most efficiently, expeditiously and completely obtained by members of the child's social world. There is a need to train Blacks, Hispanics, and former IV drug users for data collection and analysis. The work would have an authenticity that is now lacking in most of the psychosocial research on AIDS in these populations.

CONCLUSIONS

The year is 2001. A child dies. How will the staff deal with the other children who know the deceased? It is hoped that they will be able to speak to the child openly, honestly, meaningfully, addressing the needs and concerns as the child presents them. The staff will be able to do so if, over the next few years, we direct our efforts to examining the changes that have taken place in the population of dying children and in the medical community, and then consider the impact that these changes have had on the patient, family, and staff.

We need to know more about parents, well siblings, peers, and staff than we know now. We need to know their views, expectations, sources of hope, and strain at various points in the illness. More specifically, we need close study of the problems that come from living with catastrophic illnesses and how people handle these problems in the course of everyday life.

Learning what we need to learn to better care for children with AIDS is probably the most challenging of all the items on the research agenda for children with catastrophic illnesses. Here it is essential to enlist support from the Black and Hispanic community, in ways that we have not done in previous social science research.

In short, if we are to provide an atmosphere where children can freely exchange thoughts and feelings, we need a more complete understanding of the social worlds of seriously ill children than we now have and we need to give that information to the adults in the child's world – parents, staff, and teachers. Armed with the necessary information, we can effectively meet the challenges of 2001.

REFERENCES

Bluebond-Langner, Myra, D. Perkel, T. Goertzel. 1991. Pediatric cancer patients' peer relationships: The impact of an oncology camp experience. *Journal of Psychosocial Oncology*, 9(2):67-80.

Bluebond-Langner, Myra, D. Perkel, T. Goertzel. 1990. Children's knowledge of cancer and its treatment: The impact of an oncology camp experience. *Journal of Pediatrics*, 116(2):207-214.

Preventing Suicide: The State-of-the-Art

David Lester

In this paper the efforts which have been made in recent years to prevent suicide are reviewed, and suggestions are given for how suicidologists may identify new strategies for preventing suicide from those working on other public health problems. In seeking to prevent suicide, the attack can be divided into three traditionally different goals: primary, secondary, and tertiary prevention.

PRIMARY PREVENTION

Primary prevention involves the prevention of the *development* of suicidal tendencies in the society and in the individual. If suicide were preventable in this way, people in the society would never become suicidal. This is, of course, the most difficult kind of prevention. It presupposes that the causes of suicide are known which is doubtful even after these many years of scientific study. However, some suggestions can be made.

Since a large proportion of suicides are psychiatrically disturbed, the primary prevention of psychiatric disturbance would go far toward preventing suicide. The same holds true for alcoholism and drug abuse. This, though, changes the problem to that of how can we prevent people from becoming psychiatrically disturbed or substance abusers.

Barraclough (1972) examined 100 cases of completed suicide and found that 64 had depressive illnesses. Of these, 44 had experi-

David Lester, PhD, is Professor of Psychology, Richard Stockton State College, Pomona, NJ.

enced previous depressive episodes, and 21 of these met a strict criteria for a diagnosis of "recurrent affective illness." Barraclough noted that the suicide rate might have been reduced by 21 percent if these patients had been given lithium carbonate. Barraclough argued, therefore, for good diagnostic practices and the prescription of effective medication as a way of preventing suicide. Thus, use of modern medications and techniques of psychotherapy should reduce the risk of suicide in psychiatrically disturbed individuals.

Primary prevention also might focus on providing good general mental health services for communities. Ratcliffe (1962) noted that changing Dingleton Mental Hospital from a locked-ward to an open-door system of patient management was accompanied by a drop of about 60 percent in the number of suicides in the surrounding community during the following 10 years (while the suicide rate in Scotland as a whole stayed constant). Ratcliffe suggested that the open-door policy had induced more of the psychiatrically disturbed citizens in the community to use the psychiatric facility. However, no such drop in the suicide rate was noted by Walk (1967) when a community mental health center was opened in Chichester, England, and so much more research is needed to identify what factors may affect the success of such programs.

There are several groups at high risk for suicide, and early intervention with these groups might prevent suicide. For example, in the United States there recently has been a tremendous growth in groups for the close relatives and loved-ones of those who have completed suicide. Work with these survivors of suicide promises to be a potentially powerful way of preventing suicide.

More specific proposals can be made. For example, it has been found that loss of a parent during the ages of 6 to 14 is especially common in later suicides (Lester, 1989a). If children who suffer such a loss were identified, perhaps at their schools, and given appropriate psychotherapy, their potential suicidal tendencies might be defused. Other childhood trauma, such as physical and sexual abuse, has been linked to later suicides. Children subjected to these assaults also could benefit from adequate psychotherapy.

In addition, some suicide prevention workers are focusing on the research findings that suicidal tendencies are associated with low self-esteem and poor interpersonal skills. Thus, they are introducing into the schools programs whose goals are to improve the self-esteem of children and teach them better coping skills (Stivers, 1991).

In general then, any program in a society which improves the overall psychological health of its members may well prevent suicide and, we might note, other psychological and behavioral problems, too. It is hoped that, in the future our understanding of suicide will increase so that we can make many more specific proposals for the primary prevention of suicide. These school programs would seem to be more useful than those which seek merely to inform students and teachers about the clues to suicide and how to intervene with potentially suicidal individuals (Ryerson, 1991).

There is a need for caution here. Certain ways of changing society or parental behavior in order to prevent suicide might lead to alternative social and personal problems. For example, suppose that equality for females eventually raises their suicide rate to that of males. Should we, therefore, not strive for equality? Or, if a lack of external restraints on behavior leads to suicide while their presence leads to homicide, as Henry and Short (1954) have argued, to change society so as to reduce suicide may lead to an increase in homicide.

ASSESSMENT

In order to effectively work to prevent potential suicides, it is important that suicidologists improve their ability to predict suicide. We need to identify those with a high suicide risk at the societal level (by monitoring changing suicide trends in nations), the social level (by monitoring suicidal trends in group such as the elderly, the divorced, and migrants), and at the individual level (by improving the psychological tests which predict individual suicidal risk).

SECONDARY PREVENTION

Secondary prevention is early intervention with persons who are on the verge of suicide. Several strategies have been developed for this.

Suicide Prevention Centers

Suicide prevention centers have been set up in many countries in the world, and many countries have extensive networks of centers so that an individual always has a center near at hand. Suicide prevention centers typically have a 24-hour telephone crisis counseling service staffed by paraprofessional volunteers. Some centers have, in addition, walk-in clinics, and emergency outreach teams who can visit distressed individuals in the community.

This type of suicide prevention has been oriented around a crisis model of the suicidal process. People who are suicidal are conceptualized as being in a time-limited crisis state. Immediate crisis counseling will help the suicidal individual through the suicidal crisis, whereupon a normal life may resume.

Suicide prevention centers are well equipped for secondary prevention. However, as noted elsewhere, (Lester, 1989b), current suicide prevention efforts essentially are passive. A suicidal person has to contact the suicide prevention center. Active methods, such as seeking out discharged psychiatric patients, elderly males living alone, and other high risk groups must be initiated. In addition, physicians as well as community workers such as police officers, clergy, lawyers, and perhaps groups such as bartenders, prostitutes, and hair dressers who also come into contact with the public, must be sensitized to the detection of depressed, disturbed, and suicidal people.

Although early studies failed to demonstrate the impact of suicide prevention centers on the national suicide rate in England (Barraclough et al., 1977) and in the United States (Lester, 1974), more recent studies have shown a preventive effect for suicide prevention centers (Miller et al., 1984).

Restricting Access to Lethal Methods for Suicide

Clarke and Lester (1989) have argued that restricting access to lethal methods for suicide might well reduce the suicide rate. They noted that this idea first gained prominence after the reduction in the English suicide rate by about a third in the 1960s and 1970s when domestic gas was detoxified by switching from coal gas (which contains carbon monoxide) to natural gas (which does not). They conducted a number of studies to show that the availability of firearms, toxic car exhaust, and toxic domestic gas appears to be related strongly to the use of those methods for suicide, and that reducing the easy availability of these methods for suicide often reduced the overall suicide rate since not everyone switches methods for suicide when their preferred method becomes less easily available.

Clarke and Lester (1989) urged the detoxification of domestic gas, limits on the sale and ownership of firearms, restricting the size of medication prescriptions, placing the pills in plastic blisters which are hard to open, adding vomiting-inducing chemicals to medications so that an overdose will result in expulsion of the medication, prescription of suppositories rather than orally-taken tablets, prescribing the less toxic medications, cleaning up car emissions, changing the shape of the exhaust pipe to make it difficult to attach tubing, having an automatic engine turn-off mechanism if the car idles for more than a few minutes, fencing in bridges and high buildings from which people jump, and restricting the easy availability of herbicides and insecticides in developing countries. It is worth noting that removing the means for suicide is a common strategy for hospitals and prisons in their efforts to prevent patients and inmates from committing suicide.

Medical Emergency Services

Diggory (undated) has argued that we are preventing suicides with our emergency medical procedures. He estimated that in 1971, for example, the suicide rate in Pittsburgh, Pennsylvania, was reduced from 15.2 to 12.5 (a reduction of 18 percent) simply by saving the lives of those who had attempted suicide. Thus, the improvement in emergency medical care in recent years probably has increased the extent to which those who might have died in the past from their suicidal actions now survive.

TERTIARY PREVENTION

Tertiary prevention is the prevention of the recurrence of suicidal behavior in those who already have been suicidal. Strictly speaking there is no tertiary prevention for completed suicide. A completed suicide is dead. We can help only those who are not yet dead by their own hand.

However, if we bear in mind that some people who seriously intend to kill themselves are thwarted by the intervention of others and by emergency medical treatment, then we can talk about preventing the recurrence of completed suicide in these individuals. On the other hand, such individuals constitute the group which we label attempted suicides or parasuicides. Tertiary prevention, then, would involve distinguishing carefully between those who are making suicidal gestures and those who would have died but for intervention. This latter group, once identified, could be made the target population for intensive tertiary prevention efforts.

Available research shows that psychiatric treatment may be beneficial here. Montgomery and Montgomery (1982) identified three methodologically sound studies of the effects of counseling on suicidal behavior and found that only one of these indicated that counseling had a significant impact on suicidal behavior. Further research on tertiary prevention should focus on which treatments and therapies would be most effective for treating seriously suicidal people who have made lethal attempts to kill themselves.

One other suggestion for tertiary prevention would be to investigate the environments into which these lethal attempters are released. Does their environment contain suicidogenic stresses, hostile significant others who increase the likelihood of self-destructive desires, or lethal means for suicide? One suicide prevention center in the United States used to search the homes of attempted suicides, removing all guns, large knives, poisons, and lethal drugs. They were able to do this, of course, only for attempted suicides who contacted them, and they did it with the tolerance of the local police force. It is not a technique that is likely to be available to most preventers of suicide, but it does illustrate a technique for tertiary prevention.

A Source for New Strategies

Lester (1990) noted that those concerned with other types of public health and social problems have employed different strategies than those used by suicidologists. He suggested that we might profitably examine some of their strategies to see if they have potential use in preventing suicide.

Primary Prevention Strategies

An examination of the public education programs for AIDS and drug abuse reveals a very different style from that used for preventing suicide. Whereas the suicide prevention programs discuss the identification of warning signs of suicide and techniques for counseling the suicidal person, drug education programs use much more forceful and frightening techniques. For example, Yul Bryner, the American film star, recorded a video message in the weeks prior to his death from cancer urging, "Don't smoke!" which was aired on television after his death.

Suicide prevention techniques based on this viewpoint might emphasize the possibilities of disfigurement and long-term physical disability after an unsuccessful suicide attempt as well as the pain experienced by survivors of a suicide. (In this context, Frierson and Lippman [1990] recently have reported an incidence of 15 percent for colostomies after self-inflicted gunshot wounds, 6 percent for organic brain syndromes, 5 percent for seizures and 4 percent for amputations.) The various religious and moral authorities, many of whom hold suicide to be a sin, could come out as strongly opposed to suicide as they do for other life-and-death issues such as abortion.

Crime and delinquency prevention programs have realized that deviant individuals often are members of a deviant subculture who have failed to achieve success through socially-approved channels. Prevention programs have tried to draw these individuals into the larger community so that they become more socialized and in that they can achieve success through legitimate channels by, for example, giving them job training. We might adopt similar tactics for suicide prevention. It is well documented that suicide rates are higher among the unemployed (Platt, 1984), and so an obvious tactic to prevent suicide would be to help the unemployed find satisfying work. Thus, programs which draw the members of deviant subcultures into schools and colleges and into community organizations would go far in preventing suicide as well as other deviant styles of adaptation, such as drug abuse and delinquency.

Social control theories of crime focus on the social bonds and internal controls which prevent people from committing criminal acts. Criminologists argued that increasing the social bonding of people in the community would weaken their criminal tendencies. Lester (1990) argued that suicidal individuals, too, often are poorly integrated socially and have limited social networks. The major sociological theory of suicide (Durkheim, 1897), proposed that social integration and social regulation, in moderation, both served to make suicide less likely. Thus, increased social bonding should make suicides less likely. Psychological theories of suicide, too, have recognized the importance of social bonds—good relationships with parents, spouse and lovers, children and friends.

Several possible prevention techniques are suggested by this perspective. First, primary prevention could be advanced by promoting social bonding in the community and in institutions such as schools. Although such programs will never be initiated simply to prevent suicide, the effects of such programs may be widespread, decreasing involvement in all types of deviant behavior, including drug abuse and delinquency.

From an individual point of view, family therapy would appear to be the *sine qua non* for helping the suicidal individual, but it often is difficult to motivate the whole family to seek therapy. Group therapy also may be useful, but the social control perspective for suicide suggests the usefulness of social networking groups for suicidal individuals, that is, groups whose function would be to provide social experiences for the members, thereby building up their social ties.

A social conflict theory of suicide in which suicide is viewed as the result of oppression of one group in society by another group has been suggested (Lester, 1990). Evidence was produced which suggested the role suicide plays in manipulating the power balance in their relationships by oppressed individuals. It was suggested that modernization along capitalist lines might increase the risk of suicide, but the evidence for this was not yet strong. However, Hendin (1969) has argued that the oppression resulting from racism and social class may play a role in the high rates of suicide in young urban black males. Primary suicide prevention in this perspective would involve reducing the oppression in people's lives, both from the larger social forces and from individual interpersonal relationships.

Secondary Prevention Strategies

Lester (1990) also proposed a social reaction or labeling theory of suicide which focused on the ways in which people are labeled as "suicidal" in society and how they might react to this labeling. Do they reject it or do they accept it and enter the career of being suicidal? It was noted that putting patients on suicide alert in institutions (in order to monitor them more closely so as to prevent suicide) may result in labeling (Pauker and Cooper, 1990). Similarly, this could happen when people decide to call a suicide prevention center, thereby increasing their suicidal tendencies. Suicide education programs, especially in schools, may introduce people to the suicidal career and show them how to proceed in that career.

Prevention in this perspective would involve diversion, that is, treatment of the suicidal person without labeling them as suicidal. The naming of those clinics which are set up to help suicidal people may be critical, and "crisis service" may be better than "suicide prevention center" as a name. General psychological health programs in school may be more appropriate than programs that focus on suicide.

It clearly has been demonstrated that media publicity about the suicides of famous persons results in an immediate increase in the suicide rate for the next week at least (Stack, 1990). Thus, care should be taken by the media in how they present news about suicides so that learning is minimized. For example, publishing details of the method used and how it was obtained is dangerous. Glamorizing the suicide is likely to increase the suggestive impact of the suicide on others. Furthermore, researchers in the field have suggested that the media should always accompany suicide stories with information about suicide prevention resources in the community.

DISCUSSION

The major thrust of this article has been that suicidologists should broaden their approach to suicide prevention by examining the techniques used by those concerned with other public health problems such as AIDS, anti-smoking campaigns, and the prevention of drug abuse. Often workers in those areas have employed very different strategies from those used by suicide prevention workers, strategies which we should explore to see if they have potential for preventing suicide.

The programs from other public health problems often have been much more forceful than those used for suicide prevention, and much more effort has been put into primary prevention, especially improving the community so that adolescents in the community do not choose to enter upon the life paths that will lead them to deviant and disturbed life styles. We have much to learn from these programs.

REFERENCES

Barraclough, B.M. 1972. Suicide prevention, recurrent affective disorder and lithium. *British Journal of Psychiatry*, 121, 391-392.

Barraclough, B.M., C. Jennings, and J.R. Moss. 1977. Suicide prevention by the Samaritans. *Lancet*, i, 237-239.

Clarke, R.V., and D. Lester. 1989. *Suicide: Closing the Exits*. New York: Springer-Verlag.

Diggory, J. (undated). Empirical evidence for the improved prediction and prevention of suicide. Pittsburgh: Chatham College.

Durkheim, E. 1897. *Le Suicide*. Paris: Felix Alcan.

Frierson, R.L., and S.B. Lippman. 1990. Psychiatric consultation for patients with self-inflicted gunshot wounds. *Psychosomatics*, 31(1), 67-74.

Hendin, H. 1969. *Black Suicide*. New York: Basic.

Henry, A.F., and J.F. Short. 1954. *Suicide and Homicide*. New York: Free Press.

Lester, D. 1974. Effect of suicide prevention centers on suicide rates in the United States. *Health Services Reports*, 89, 37-39.

Lester, D. 1989a. Experience of personal loss and later suicide. *Acta Psychiatrica Scandinavica*, 79, 450-452.

Lester, D. 1989b. *Can We Prevent Suicide*? New York: AMS.

Lester, D. 1990. *Understanding and Preventing Suicide: New Perspectives*. Springfield, IL: Charles Thomas.

Miller, H., D. Coombs, J. Leeper, and S. Barton. 1984. An analysis of the effects of suicide prevention facilities on suicide rates in U.S. *American Journal of Public Health*, 74, 340-343.

Montgomery, S., and D. Montgomery. 1982. Drug treatment of suicidal behavior. *Advances in Biochemistry & Psychopharmacology*, 32, 347-355.

Pauker, S.L., and A.M. Cooper. Paradoxical patient reactions to psychiatric life support. *American Journal of Psychiatry*, 147, 488-491.

Platt, S. 1984. Unemployment and suicidal behavior. *Social Science & Medicine*, 19, 93-115.

Ratcliffe, R.W. 1962. The open door. *Lancet*, ii, 188-190.

Ryerson, D. 1991. Suicide awareness education in schools. In A.A. Leenaars & S. Wenckstern (eds.), *Suicide Prevention in Schools*. New York: Hemisphere, 99-112.

Stack, S. 1990. Media impacts on suicide. In D. Lester (ed.) *Current Concepts of Suicide*. Philadelphia: The Charles Press, Publishers, 107-120.

Stivers, C. 1991. Promotion of self-esteem in the prevention of suicide. In A.A. Leenaars & S. Wenckstern (eds.), *Suicide Prevention in Schools*. New York: Hemisphere, 51-69.

Walk, D. 1967. Suicide and community care. *British Journal of Psychiatry*, 113, 1381-1391.

Thanatology: Wither Thou Goest?

Allen P. Fertziger

It is now three decades since the revolutionary pioneers of what would become the discipline of Thanatology spoke out against the destructive denial of death that had reached insufferable proportions in health care. Three decades have passed since the forceful words and deeds of such figures as Feifel (1959), Kübler-Ross (1969), and Kutscher (1960) transformed our understanding and treatment of the terminally ill and their loved ones. And yet, in spite of all of that Thanatology has done for the dying, their loved ones, and the bereaved; in spite of all the professional thanatological organizations that now exist; in spite of all our scholarly inquiry and research; and in spite of all of the courses now routinely taught on this subject, thanatologists continue to function as a largely misunderstood group of professional "outsiders" whose seeming fascination with death, loss, and human suffering remains enigmatic and counter-current to the mainstream of cure-oriented health care.

Still, the seeds of compassionate care, courage, and determination to meet death on its own terms, so forcefully planted by our pioneering founders, have now clearly begun to germinate, and give every indication of continued growth. But the larger professional community whose task it is to tend to these delicate seedlings seems, to this observer at least, to be intent on cultivating Thanatology in separate and somewhat exclusive professional gardens of bounded professional turf.

The National Congress of Thanatology (1990) came at a remarkable time, and thus provided those of us in the field of Thanatology

---

Allen P. Fertziger, PhD, Chevy Chase, MD.

with a rare opportunity to begin to balance the natural professional tendency to divide and specialize. The Congress was an opportunity to come together in a spirit of union seeking to forge the new linkages and commonalities that will bind us in the future. It also was an opportunity to begin to give shape to the professional vision from which the activity of the years ahead will take form.

DEATH: THE GREAT LEVELLER ALSO CAN BE THE GREAT UNIFIER

Twenty-five hundred years ago, Socrates was preparing to die at the hands of the leaders of Athens. He urged his students and followers to remember that "the true philosopher studies to die, and to him of all men is death least terrible." It is often difficult, perhaps impossible, for those outside of Thanatology to understand that what appears to be a fascination with "death and dying" is, in truth, a reflection of a deeper, spiritual commitment to "life and living." Ours is a discipline that is as much concerned with the state and fate of the soul as we are with the body. We struggle in trying to explain how our goal to be health providers for whom "death is least terrible" is not simply to dwell on death, pain, and unavoidable suffering, but to redefine these inevitable clinical outcomes into therapeutic agendas of greater effectiveness.

Though modern society, for all our science and technology, is no closer than Socrates to finding a solution to the riddle of death, we in Thanatology are well positioned to working with the deeper symbolic significance of death. There may be no "answer," but that hardly means nothing can be done other than denial and ignorance. Additionally, we in Thanatology are bound by a common desire, a collective readiness, and a professional ability to answer the call of human beings found with seemingly insoluble human dilemmas.

It is the very insolubility which death symbolizes to society that is the bond holding the thanatological community together. We share in common a spirit that will not be deterred from joining another in pain and suffering—simply because we lack the correct "answer" or the suitable methodology, or a guarantee of success. Though this essential thanatological spirit of unconditionally serving the suffering is timeless. We now stand at a moment in human history where the need for a clear collective thanatological mind and voice is crucial. Never before has our collective hubris left us so divided and at the edge of a terrifying despair. The ecological health of our planet is endangered as never before; impossible wars and political chaos is omni-present; and whole systems and civilizations seem poised precipices of despair. Is it not ironic that at precisely such a time of scientific and medical "progress," human suffering is so great? The thanatological community has the ability to both understand and to heal this modern madness, but first we will have to learn how to speak as one voice and learn to act as one body.

We, in Thanatology, cannot afford to forget that our profession was born only after the neglect and the denial of the dying and their families, though invisible to others, became apparent to us. It was as if the collective eyes of Thanatology could see what the eyes of other competent and caring professionals could not. All of our progress and professionalization notwithstanding, that very condition still prevails today. Yes, we have hospices, terminal care, and a widespread awareness of the stages of grief. But the very same dynamic that allowed previously workable agendas to obscure human suffering thirty years ago is still alive and well today in the 1990s. Different forms and situations, perhaps, but the very same scenarios of human suffering are being played out unwittingly by those too attached to therapeutic traditions that now hurt where once they helped. We, in Thanatology, understand this peculiar and improbable health care dynamic, and are obliged to cultivate the vision and the voice that will be increasingly needed in the days to come. Yes, there are journals, professional organizations, a vital hospice movement, and many more palpable signs of thanatological progress. But these are still only the small germinating plants of the thanatological movement; they are not the garden which we must recognize is ours to envision and develop. Much fertile land remains to be cultivated, and many humanizing seeds need to be planted.

Death always can be relied upon to push us to our limits. Socrates and a timeless philosophical tradition have shown us how death is both, literally and figuratively, the "final frontier." As the privileged profession among the health scientists who are the guardians of this extraordinary human frontier, we must stand united with a vigilance to guard against the denial of death wherever its hydra-like head is bound to appear. This united vigilance, along with cultivating all of the seeds we have planted, also must become a central element in our link of unity.

NECESSARY GENERALISTS IN A WORLD OF SPECIALISTS

I have spent many hours in lecture halls, reflecting on how minimally attended were many varied and always fascinating thanatological discussions. Despite the bustling activity that feverishly went on around us, I was always struck by how invisible thanatological meetings seemed to be. It was apparent that we were discussing topics which had great bearing on many of the issues which deeply concerned medicine and health care. So, why were not more of our health professional colleagues joining us in thanatological discussions that seemed so terribly relevant to what they were doing? Were we too "philosophical"? Were we too vague or unscientific? Was it that we were unclear? In time, however, the answer has become more clear; thanatologists were approaching the very same issues that other health care providers were addressing, but were doing so as "generalists." Our concern is one that goes out in ever widening spheres of interest. More often than not, their concern converges in a focus of high intensity. While they were examining narrower and narrower issues of relevance, thanatologists were addressing wider and wider issues that involved not only the patient, but the family, the community, and even the well-being of the caregiver. Though Thanatology need not be general, and can obviously address highly specialized issues, it is important for us to understand that there is a very strong component of "generalist" at the core of the discipline. It is important to acknowledge this central difference: this is not to say that specialists are better or worse than generalists, but to acknowledge that the care of human beings deserves a healthy balance of these two useful, but very different perspectives.

As it is with almost every aspect of life, it is the "nuts and bolts" that demand so much of our attention, so that we almost never have time to take stock of the "whole picture." This is what makes Thanatology such a special discipline at this time. It is true that our propensity to look at the "whole picture" renders us somewhat out of it, at a time when most every other health professional seems intent on focusing in on a specific "part." But it also is precisely this ability to remain steadfast in our interest on holistic issues that makes Thanatology so important today. Our perspective uniquely qualifies us to function collectively as a sort of quasi-health professional conscience. Our vigilance for emerging and otherwise invisible forms of human suffering permits us to readily and clearly see when a once effective treatment may unexpectedly become worse than the disease being treated. Furthermore, it is our propensity and ability to look at death straight on that can enable us to attend to a patient's "soul"—a long respected human entity that has tended to be much maligned and neglected in these scientific materialist times.

Whether our concern is with a terminal or a chronic illness or whether it is with the grief of lost life, organ, or a loved one, what makes thanatologists unique is our willingness to assume the widest and most holistic posture available. Whether it involves the issues surrounding something as concrete as respiratory therapy or as abstract as cross-cultural perspectives on loss, where we are unique is in our willingness to enter any spiritual or material world on behalf of those we serve. It is this very holistic perspective that makes Thanatology so deeply rewarding and yet makes thanatologists seem so strange and alien to the mainstream of other health professions. Moreover, the future of Thanatology will stand on our ability to maintain our balance on this subtle professional distinction.

Can we continue resisting the temptation to become yet another "specialist" in a health professional sea of specialists? Can we attend to the patient's spiritual soul in an atmosphere that most assuredly prefers to treat the body alone? Can we maintain the essential bridges that keep us connected to our medical scientific colleagues? These are crucial questions.

PAIN, SUFFERING, AND CONSCIENCE – MODERN PHYSICIANS OF THE SOUL

The tendency to specialize in health care is closely linked to the philosophy of materialism that quite naturally tends to reduce the whole individual to constituent parts. For all its brilliance and productivity, this scientific reductionism has tended to strip human beings bare of their soul. The very "soul" that has for so long formed the basis of our Judeo-Christian civilization has now been reduced literally to something akin to a psychological function that (in the words of modern science) will one day be localized in some brain structure. For those of us in Thanatology, however, the inner world of the individual and the world of his or her soul is not where our work ends, but where it begins. The diagnostic reality which we in Thanatology have labored so long and hard to create, that is "terminal illness," is one that literally frees the dying patient from an agenda focused on "healing the body" to one that can begin to "heal the soul" – at its most profound crisis.

Under this banner of what was once called "healing the soul," we in Thanatology have, in effect, been building a professional discipline. We have, if you will, been given the license to attend to a full spectrum of spiritual (i.e., non-organic/non-curing) phenomena. Yet, we recognize that "healing the soul" is an activity that need not and should not be restricted to life's final moments. Just as we must be vigilant to emergent suffering from the most unlikely places, so, too, must we be vigilant to see where our health care system compromises our spiritual well-being at times other than death. Thanatology is, to be sure, about AIDS. But also it is about the experience of loss in the most generic sense. It is as much about the more chronic aspects of aging and other afflictions of life's final passage as it is about hospice and the acute phase of dying. It is as much about understanding cross-cultural perspectives of loss and grief as it is about healing injuries and human suffering that comes in the wake of a severing of the human-animal bond.

As we in the Thanatology community look to the future, let us temporarily lose our hold on the hard earned arenas of expertise and achievement. Let us do this long enough not only so we can see the enormous work that lies ahead, but so that we can recognize the rare privilege of sharing in this demanding and challenging professional opportunity.

REFERENCES

Feifel, Herman. 1959. *The Meaning of Death*. New York: McGraw-Hill Book Company.

First National Congress of Thanatology. 1990. (September 13-15). New York: Columbia-Presbyterian Medical Center.

Kübler-Ross, Elisabeth. 1969. *On Death and Dying*. New York: The Macmillan Company.

Kutscher, Austin. 1960. *Death and Bereavement*. Springfield, IL: Charles C Thomas Publisher.

What Should a Thanatology Organization Do?

Harold B. Haley

The concept of a National Association of Thanatology Organizations (NATO) deserves serious consideration. Several aspects present themselves:

1. What are possible advantages and disadvantages of (or reasons for and against) such an association?
2. What should the nature and structure be?
3. What should be its functions?

Each of these aspects will have different components with differing importance, priorities and do-ability. Following are some thoughts on these issues.

SHOULD THERE BE A NATO?

The current status of thanatology points up a number of needs that a NATO could meet. Two appear to be particularly important: one is internal within the thanatology community; the other is in relationship with the broader society.

The tremendous increase in attention to death, dying, and bereavement in the past decade has increased greatly the involvement of professionals in many different disciplines and has logarithmically increased the types and levels of problems and target audiences. We have no idea of what is being lost by the limited communication among the various professionals in the field and between

---

Harold B. Haley, MD, is Clinical Professor of Surgery, Baylor College of Medicine, Houston, TX.

the professionals and society as a whole. We need to learn from each other, work with each other, and increase all levels of communication.

A vital role for NATO is to serve as a visible presence for thanatology interests to the general public, governments, and other communities, such as the academic. An application of this is the public expression of an organized thanatology opinion on specific subjects, e.g., the various states consider and pass legislation such as natural death acts. There are other applications: (1) Research and education needs are many. Communication, cooperation and organization would further these areas; (2) A central database would be an aspect of this; (3) The professional field needs development. Identification of people and resources in the various organizations and disciplines would add to the efficacy of all. Definition of fields and subfields would lead to development of standards, training programs, and certification. This could include development, identification, and hiring procedures for people working in thanatology.

An overall approach to serving the membership of the various organizations could result in joint projects in research and education. This could be applied to identification of different target populations and the development of projects for appropriate groups. International and cross-cultural areas would benefit from organized attention.

Discussion of reasons to have NATO must include consideration of major problems and negative factors. A successful NATO will require dedicated people, significant time and effort, and effective funding. Defined and accepted objectives are essential. Mutuality of interests, recognition of each others' roles and concerns, and functioning together by such diverse professionals may be difficult to achieve.

NATURE AND STRUCTURE OF A NATO

The concept of an organization of organizations raises many questions. What organizations? There should be formal organizations with defined membership, structure, and mission. At the beginning there should be a temporary organizing group to establish criteria and evaluate proposed member groups. Deliberate effects should be made to include groups with thanatology interests from a wide spectrum of intellectual, professional, religious, political, and ethnic beliefs.

Officers, structure, and procedures that are common to all groups would be needed. An assembly of organization representatives would have ultimate authority, which would have to be confirmed by the parent organizations. Problems are inevitable because of time lags between NATO resolutions and meetings of parent organizations which could be lengthy. The NATO would need a small executive committee to make and carry out policies between annual meetings of the NATO or possibly more frequent meetings of a Board of Directors. Parent organizations also might need an executive committee with authority to act on NATO affairs. As a start, parent organizations should have one representative and possibly an alternate. Later, consideration might be given to some sort of proportional representation.

There is a series of related starting questions. Where would the organization be based? Who would write the constitution, by-laws, and procedures? How would staff, ex-officio members, duration of offices and representatives holding their positions be determined? Can a mechanism be developed for formal participation by individuals? For example, some parent organizations may rotate representatives, but in time, might have ex-representatives who still could make significant contributions. It also is likely that there are contributing persons without an organizational affiliation. It might be possible to have an organization of individuals that could then have a representative to the NATO. Non-representing persons also could serve on sub-groups.

Many sub-groups would be needed. Some of these might include standing and ad hoc committees, and special interest groups (SIGS). Obvious committees include: membership, publications, fiscal and audit, meeting planning, legislative, and education and research. Both cross- and intradisciplinary groups may be indicated.

Start-up would require outside funding as NATO would probably not be financially self-sustaining initially. A NATO would be best as a free-standing organization, but could get a start by being affiliated with another group.

FUNCTIONS

What could and should a NATO do? As noted earlier, there is the need for wide and deep communication among thanatology professionals, and a recognition of the importance of a thanatology presence to external society.

There is unlimited opportunity to improve and increase communication and, thus, add to learning and skills, ultimately making all groups more effective. Communication methods would include: newsletters for rapid presentation of information, calls for action (this should be started immediately); later, a journal of the organization itself or an affiliation with a journal in the field; an annual meeting with a wide range of activities; and much personal interaction on group or one-to-one bases. Special projects, such as emphasizing roles for minority group professionals and participating in cross-cultural studies, are possible. Communication functions should be general and cross-disciplinary, but there also should be very specific functions by SIGS or committees. Examples of these would be monitoring and reporting legal adjudications involving thanatology. Cross-disciplinary task forces and working groups could provide communicative learning for all concerned.

The role of presence has many facets. National legislation can be actively influenced by testifying before congressional committees, or by NATO representatives meeting with the staff people of senators and congresspersons. NATO could designate members of the parent organizations to express their views to both executive and legislative governmental branches. All of this also could apply equally to state governments. A consistent and active presence could provide thanatology education to academic and professional organizations. Another major role would be to present thanatological viewpoints to national and local media.

There are other important functions. Formal studies could be performed to identify and define needs in thanatology for research, educational, political, or organizational activities. Some of these studies should be an early-on activity of NATO. A major ongoing function should be to significantly expand the quality and quantity of research in thanatology. Seminars, Delphi studies, and other means to generate and stimulate research activities should be encouraged. Cooperative group studies, multidisciplinary studies, better methodologies, education in research techniques, help in fundraising, help in reporting, and, especially, dissemination of research results are other needed functions. At a later point there may be a place for the development of advocacy programs.

This essay is only a beginning. It is hoped it will be a starting point and will stimulate others to give their thoughts about a National Association of Thanatology Organizations.

APPENDIX

Members of the 1st National Congress of Thanatology

National Chairperson

Dr. Samuel C. Klagsbrun

Liaison Chairpersons

Dr. John D. Morgan
Dr. Vanderlyn Pine
Dr. Richard Ellis

Keynote Speaker

Dr. Herman Feifel

Coordinator

Dr. Elizabeth J. Clark

Secretary

Dr. Austin H. Kutscher

Executive Planning Committee

Dr. Jeanne Quint Benoliel
Dr. Sandra Bertman
Dr. Andrew Blitzer
Dr. Myra Bluebond-Langner
Dr. John Bruhn
Dr. Dana Cable
Dr. Charles A. Corr
Dr. Bruce Danto
Dr. Ben Dickerson
Dr. Kenneth Doka
Dr. Robert Fulton
Dr. Ivan K. Goldberg
Dr. Ida Martinson
Dr. David Meagher
Jane Nichols
Dr. Therese Rando
Dr. William Regelson
Dr. Victor Scalise
Dr. Irene B. Seeland
Dr. Florence E. Selder
Dr. Phyllis Silverman
Dr. Robert G. Stevenson
Dr. Judith Stillion
Dr. Leslie M. Thompson

Dr. Therese Goodrich
Dr. Earl Grollman
Dr. Harold B. Haley
Dr. Hannah Hedrick
William V. Hocker
Dr. Dennis Klass
Dr. Gilbert Kliman
Madeline E. Lambrecht, MSN, RN
Dr. David Lester
Dr. Dorothy C.H. Ley
Dr. Alan Lyall
Dr. Richard Torpie
Dr. Mary Vachon
Todd Van Beck, MA
Florence Wald, MN, MS
Henry Wald
Dr. Hannelore Wass
Dr. Avery D. Weisman
Rev. William Wendt, STD
Dr. David Wollner
Dr. J. William Worden

Planning Committee Members

Ruth Abrams, MSW
Denyse Adler, MA
Marcia Alig
Dr. Thomas Attig
Dr. Rochelle Balter
Dr. Michael Bartalos
Georganna Beffa, RN, MS
Dr. Robert Bendiksen
Dr. D. Peter Birkett
Dr. Wilma Bulkin
Penelope Buschman, RN, MS
Dr. Arthur C. Carr
Dr. Daniel J. Cherico
Dr. James S. Cimino
Christopher S. Clason
Susan J. Cohen, CSW, ACSW
Dr. Francine Cournos
Dr. Alice Cullinan
Dr. Robert DeBellis
Dr. Ann de Jong
Herman de Mönnink
Lois Chapman Dick, ACSW
Carol Farkas, RN, MPH
Dr. Tamara Ferguson
Dr. Allen P. Fertziger
Marcia Fishman, RN, MA
Dr. Mark Flapan
Paula Fogelberg, LCSW
Dr. Richard B. Freeman
Carole Lambert, MPA
Claire F. Leach, MSS
Dr. Dan Leviton
Dr. Randall Lockwood
Edward Madera
Carole G. Maeder, MSW
Dr. Ruth Malkinson
Dr. Eric R. Marcus
Dr. Otto S. Margolis
Dr. Terry Martin
Dr. Nicholas Michelli
Milton Miller, CPA
Dr. Richard Miller
Dr. Judy Oakes
Rev. Brian O'Connor
Sr. Patrice O'Connor, RN, MA
Dr. Mohamed Osman
Dr. David Peretz
Raoul I. Pinette
Dr. Larry Platt
Elizabeth R. Prichard, ACSW
F. Barbara Rabinowitz, ACSW
Howard Raether, JD
Dr. Marilyn M. Rawnsley
Dr. Patricia Rieker
Anne Rosberger, ACSW
Gerald Rosner, CLU, ChFC
Dr. Joel Savishinsky
Daniel J. Schaefer

Dr. Carole Fudin
Erna Furman
Dr. Robert Furman
Allen Glass
Sydell Glass
Dr. Allen Goldberg
Rabbi Jacob Goldberg
Dr. Meeta Goswami
Dr. Carlo E. Grossi
Roberta Halporn, MA
Jeanne Harper, MPS
Joanne Hayes, MA, RN
Dr. Frederic P. Herter
Barbara Hoffman, JD
Dr. William J. Kay
John M. Kiernan, MBA
Ann Kliman, MA
Hermine Koplin Kutscher
Lorraine Sciara, MPH, RN
Dr. Egilde Seravalli
Mary-Ellen Siegel, ACSW
Dr. Aileen Silverman
Dr. Robert Slater
Rev. Carole E. Smith-Torres
Naomi Stearns, LICSW
Dr. Irene Sullivan
Dr. Margot Tallmer
Dr. Jerrold Tannenbaum
Dr. Vamik Volkan
Janet P. Wagner
Dr. Morris Wessel
Dr. Alan D. Wolfelt
Dr. Susan Wolfelt
Dr. Ellen Zinner
Grace Zambelli, EdS, ATR

CONGRESSIONAL ADDRESSES

Opening Remarks

Florence Wald, M.N., M.S., F.A.A.N.
Clinical Professor
Yale University School of Nursing
New Haven, CT

Keynote Address

"The Thanotological Community: Respice, adspice and prospice"

Herman Feifel, Ph.D.
Chief, Psychology Service
Veterans Administration Outpatient Clinic
Los Angeles, CA

Featured Presentations

"State of the Art v. State of the Science"

Samuel C. Klagsbrun, M.D.
Associate Clinical Professor of Psychiatry
College of Physicians and Surgeons, Columbia University
Director, Four Winds Hospital
Katonah, NY

"The Needs, Goals and Direction
of the Thanatology Community"

Vanderlyn R. Pine, Ph.D.
President, Association for Death Education and Counseling
Professor of Sociology
State University of New York, New Paltz

"Undervalued Caregiving: An Issue of the Thanatology Community"

Jeanne Quint Benoliel, R.N., D.N.Sc., F.A.A.N.
Professor Emeritus of Community Health Care Systems
School of Nursing
University of Washington, Seattle

"The Implications of Professionalizing the Care of the Bereaved"

Phyllis R. Silverman, Ph.D.
Child Bereavement Study, Harvard Medical School
Department of Psychiatry, Massachusetts General Hospital
Boston, MA

"The Changing Complexion of Mourning in the 90s:
It Doesn't Look Good"

Therese A. Rando, Ph.D.
Clinical Psychologist and Clinical Director
Therese A. Rando Associates, Ltd.
Warwick, RI

"A Sociologist Looks at the AIDS Epidemic"

Robert Fulton, Ph.D.
Director, Center for Death Education and Research
Professor of Sociology
University of Minnesota
Minneapolis, MN

"The Changing Images of AIDS"

Sandra L. Bertman, Ph.D.
Director, Program of Medical Humanities
University of Massachusetts Medical Center
Worcester, MA

"Thanatology Literature: Time to Search for New Directions"

Roberta Halporn, M.A.
Director, Center for Thanatology Research and Education, Inc.
Brooklyn, NY

"Organizing the Field of Thanatology"

Harold B. Haley, M.D.
Clinical Professor of Surgery
Baylor College of Medicine
Houston, TX

"Children and Death: Issues for the 90s"

Myra Bluebond-Langner, Ph.D.
Professor of Anthropology
Rutgers University
New Brunswick, NJ

"The Funeral Industry and Thanatology"

William V. Hocker, Past-President
National Funeral Directors Association
The Loewen Group, Inc.
Burnaby, British Columbia

"Spreading Our Knowledge"

Hannelore L. Wass, Ph.D.
Professor of Educational Psychology
University of Florida
Gainesville, FL

"Educational Needs in Thanatology"

Richard R. Ellis, Ed.D.
Associate Professor of Applied Psychology
New York University
New York, NY

Planning Session Addresses

"Youth Prevention Suicide"

Jeanne M. Harper, M.P.S.
State Coordinator, Wisconsin Youth Suicide Prevention
Executive Director, Alpha-Omega Venture
Marinette, WI

"Is Suicide Prevention Possible?"

David Lester, Ph.D.
Professor of Psychology
Richard Stockton State College
Pomona, NJ

"Enhancing Services for the Dying"

Ida M. Martinson, R.N., Ph.D., F.A.A.N.
Professor of Family Health Care Nursing
University of California, San Francisco

"Gaps in Services for the Dying"

Marion B. Dolan, R.N.
President, Heritage Home Health/Heritage Hospice
Bristol, NH

"New Directions in Thanatology: Implications for Research"

Patricia P. Rieker, Ph.D.
Director of Psychosocial Research
Dana-Farber Cancer Institute
Assistant Professor, Harvard Medical School
Boston, MA

"Research Issues in Thanatology—New Directions"

Madeline E. Lambrecht, M.S.N., R.N.
Assistant Professor of Nursing
University of Delaware
Newark, DE

"Violent Death/Sudden Death/Catastrophic Death"

Bruce Danto, M.D.
Private Practice
Fullerton, CA

"Dirty Death: Are We Denying Its Existence and Avoiding Those Impacted by It?"

Lois Chapman Dick, M.A.L.S., M.S.W.
Board of Directors and Editor of *Forum*
Association for Death Education and Counseling
Kirkland, WA

"Offering Services to the Non-Traditional Groups"

Marcia F. Alig
Past-President, The Compassionate Friends, Inc.
Princeton Junction, NJ

"Enhancing Services for the Bereaved"

Ben Wolfe, M.Ed.
Board of Directors
Association for Death Education and Counseling
Program Director, St. Mary's Grief Support Center
Duluth, MN

"Adrift in a Sea of Broken Parts:
The Right Connections for a Healing Environment"

Leslie M. Thompson, Ph.D.
Dean for Graduate Studies and Research
Texas Woman's University
Denton, TX

"Unrecognized Grief"

Kenneth J. Doka, Ph.D.
Professor of Gerontology
College of New Rochelle
New Rochelle, NY

"The Concept of Pathological Grief"

Alan D. Wolfelt, Ph.D.
Director, Center for Loss and Life Transition
Fort Collins, CO

"Setting Standards: An Overview of Certification Activities in the Death-Related Fields"

Ellen S. Zinner, Psy.D.
Vice President, Association for Death Education and Counseling
Assistant Professor of Counseling
Frostburg State University, Frostburg, MD

"Setting the Standards for the Field"

David K. Meagher, Ed.D.
Associate Professor, Thanatology Program
Brooklyn College, Brooklyn, NY

"Mitigating Staff Stress: Supervisory Aspects"

Naomi M. Stearns, LICSW
Past-President, National Association for Oncology Social Workers
Director of Social Work
Dana-Farber Cancer Institute
Boston, MA

"The Process of Stress of the Caregiver's Grief"

Sally Featherstone, M.N., R.N., C.S.
Clinical Nurse Specialist
Barnes Hospital at Washington University Medical Center
St. Louis, MO

"Legal Concerns of Persons with Serious Illness: Cancer Survivors as Case Example"

Barbara Hoffman, J.D.
Senior Vice President
National Coalition for Cancer Survivorship
Cranbury, NJ

"Patients' Rights on Collision Course with Society's Best Interests?"

T. Patrick Hill, M.A.
Director of Education
Concern for Dying/Society for the Right to Die
New York, NY

"New Roles in Aging"

Tamara Ferguson, Ph.D., C.C.S.
Research Associate, Lafayette Clinic
Adjunct Associate Professor of Sociology in Psychiatry
Wayne State University School of Medicine
Detroit, MI

"Gerontological Issues in Thanatology"

Margot Tallmer, Ph.D.
Professor of Psychology
Hunter College of the City of New York, NY

"Childhood Issues of Thanatology"

Erna Furman
Cleveland Center for Research in Child Development
Cleveland, OH

"Grief in Childhood and Adolescence"

Morris A. Wessel, M.D.
Clinical Professor of Pediatrics
Yale University School of Medicine
New Haven, CT

"Death Education Across the Lifespan"

Robert G. Stevenson, Ed.D.
Instructor of Death Education Programs of River Dell High School,
Fairleigh Dickinson and Bergen Community College, NJ
Co-Chairperson, Columbia University Seminar on Death
New York, NY

"Facing the Reality of Death"

Victor F. Scalise, Jr., D. Min.
Mount Ida College-National Center for Death Education
Newton Centre, MA

"Clinical Interventions—Needs of the Discipline"

Florence Selder, R.N., Ph.D.
Associate Professor, Urban Research Center
University of Wisconsin, Milwaukee, WI

"Death: The Needs of the Survivor"

Michael K. Bartalos, M.D.
Department of Pediatrics
Columbia University, New York, NY

"Issues of Survivorship and Chronic Illness"

Alijeta Ortiz, MSW
Cancer Care, Inc.
New York, NY

Moderators/Recorders

Diane M. Ryerson, ACSW
Chair, Bergen County Task Force on Suicide Prevention
Director, South Bergen Mental Health Center, Inc.
Lyndhurst, NJ

L. Allen Haney, Ph.D., C.C.S.
Professor of Sociology
University of Houston
Houston, TX

Joanne D. Hayes, M.A., R.N.
Board Member, Oncology Nursing Society
President, The Nexus Group
Nutley, NJ

Ann de Jong Hodgson, Ph.D., R.N.
Nurse Psychotherapist
Private Practice
Montclair, NJ

Carole A. Lambert, M.P.A.
New York, NY

Anne W. Rosberger, C.S.W., A.C.S.W.
Executive Director, Bereavement and Loss Center
New York, NY

Rochelle Balter, Ph.D.
Executive Committee, American Institute of Life-Threatening Illness and Loss
Staff Therapist
Institute for Rational-Emotive Therapy
New York, NY

Thomas W. Attig, Ph.D.
Chair and Professor
Department of Philosophy
Bowling Green State University
Bowling Green, OH

Denyse Adler, M.A.
Associate Director
The Cancer Institute
New Brunswick Affiliated Hospital
New Brunswick, NJ

Paula J. Fogelberg, L.C.S.W.
Psychotherapist
Private Practice
Franklin, TN

Grace Zambelli, Ed.S., A.T.R.
Registered Art Therapist
The Hospice, Inc.
Montclair, NJ

Mary-Ellen Siegel, M.S.W., A.C.S.W.
Senior Teaching Associate
Department of Community Medicine (Social Work)
Mount Sinai School of Medicine
City University of New York, NY

Sr. Alice Cullinan, Ph.D.
Director, Newburgh Counseling Service
Newburgh, NY

Susan Slaninka, Ed.D., R.N.
Chair, Department of Nursing
West Chester University
West Chester, PA

Index